Cross-Sectional Imaging in Crohn's Disease

Jordi Rimola
Editor

Cross-Sectional Imaging in Crohn's Disease

Springer

Editor
Jordi Rimola
Department of Radiology
Hospital Clínic of Barcelona, CIBEREHD, University of Barcelona
Barcelona
Spain

ISBN 978-3-319-96585-7 ISBN 978-3-319-96586-4 (eBook)
https://doi.org/10.1007/978-3-319-96586-4

Library of Congress Control Number: 2018965474

This Springer imprint is published by the registered company Springer Nature Switzerland AG
The registered company address is: Gewerbestrasse 11, 6330 Cham, Switzerland

Preface

The length and caliber of the small bowel make it challenging to evaluate by conventional endoscopy and radiology techniques. Not long ago, barium studies were the only way to image the bowel, providing meager visualization of the lumen and mucosal irregularities. The past 15 years have seen tremendous improvements in cross-sectional imaging technologies and innovative ways to apply them in evaluating the bowel.

Cross-sectional imaging's powerful objective insights into the disease process have earned it a firm position in current diagnostic and management paradigms for inflammatory bowel disease. Clinicians dealing with inflammatory bowel disease recognize that cross-sectional imaging is the technique of choice for assessing inflammation in Crohn's disease, where transmural involvement requires more comprehensive assessment than endoscopy can offer. Similarly, in perianal disease, MRI enables clinicians to determine the optimal management strategy and to assess the efficacy of therapeutic interventions.

As guest editor, I am fortunate to have received contributions from a number of distinguished authors in inflammatory bowel disease, as well as from younger investigators with experience in the field. I am grateful to all the authors for their generous contributions in sharing their cutting-edge knowledge and expertise in the different topics. I am sure that this book will become a valuable resource for radiologists as well as for clinicians.

Barcelona, Spain — Jordi Rimola

Contents

The Clinical Impact of Cross-Sectional Imaging on Crohn's Disease Management

1

Ellen M. Zimmermann

Abstract

A new era of Crohn's disease management exists where decisions are made by objective data as a necessary adjunct to patient symptoms. Cross-sectional imaging, particularly CT enterography (CTE) and MR enterography (MRE), provides powerful objective insights into the disease process resulting in a firm place for cross-sectional imaging in our current diagnostic and management paradigms. The high sensitivity and specificity of the techniques for the presence of *bowel inflammation* have helped pinpoint the location and severity of disease enabling diagnosis and facilitating assessment of symptoms. The ability to identify disease *complications* has helped direct medical therapy and enables more robust presurgical assessment. Emerging data suggest that cross-sectional imaging findings are sensitive to changes in inflammation resulting from our potent biologic therapies and may be used in amazing new ways such as in predicting disease course. Technological advances in CT and MR enterography have provided new insights into the disease processes while enhancing patient safety and tolerability. The goal of this chapter is to provide a gastroenterologist's view of how cross-sectional imaging fits our current and future management algorithm. These remarkable technologies enable gastroenterologists and radiologists, working together, to serve our patient population in profound ways.

E. M. Zimmermann (✉)
Division of Gastroenterology, University of Florida, Gainesville, FL, USA
e-mail: ezimmer2@ufl.edu

J. Rimola (ed.), *Cross-Sectional Imaging in Crohn's Disease*,
https://doi.org/10.1007/978-3-319-96586-4_1

1.1 Disease Pathogenesis

Crohn's disease exists along with ulcerative colitis as the two major conditions under the umbrella term inflammatory bowel disease (IBD). Crohn's disease is a chronic inflammatory disease that can affect any region of the gastrointestinal tract with the distal ileum and the colon being the most commonly affected regions. The natural history of Crohn's disease is for chronic inflammation to affect the entire thickness of the bowel wall from the mucosa at the luminal interface to the serosa. Ulcerations, ranging from superficial aphthous ulcerations to deep serpiginous ulcers, are pathologic hallmarks of the disease. Chronic inflammation typified by lymphocytic infiltrates dominates the histological landscape, and the cytokines and other factors elaborated in the process of cellular interactions contribute to the pathologic findings [1, 2]. Inflammation triggers fibrotic pathways with TGFβ, PDGF, and IGF-1 and other factors playing important roles [3, 4]. As the process continues, smooth muscle in the bowel wall proliferates, and scar tissue develops with stricturing and luminal narrowing. One of the mysteries of the disease is the presence of skip lesions, that is, intensely inflamed regions separated by normal bowel. Also a mystery is why some patients, particularly young patients, develop serious Crohn's disease in multiple locations, while other patients have isolated ileal ulcers that may exist unrecognized for years. It is also unknown why some patients seem to progress to complicated disease quickly, sometimes presenting with fistulizing disease at the disease onset, whereas others may have silent disease for years. The reason for the diversity of presentation is unknown but is likely immunologically and genetically determined [3, 5]. It has recently been recognized, for example, that some of the youngest IBD patients have germ line mutations in fundamental immune pathways. In these most vulnerable patients, IBD can coexist with other autoimmune diseases [6].

The underlying etiology for Crohn's disease also remains a mystery, but research on cytokine networks and immunologic cellular interactions has provided remarkable insights into the pathogenesis [1, 2]. Genetic studies have yielded identification of mutations in over 200 contributory genes [5]. The first recognized gene association and the most robust of all the recognized risk alleles is a mutation in the gene for NOD2. NOD2 is an intracellular protein that recognizes a specific motif, muramyl dipeptide, which is a common bacterial cell wall component, peptidoglycan (PG). PG on the bacterial surface helps direct the appropriate response to bacteria by interacting with pattern recognition receptors on the surface of host immune cells [6, 7]. Recognition of the importance of the host immune-bacterial interactions opened the door for a decade of research on the microbiome that has impacted a wide range of disease processes. Research into the microbiome has highlighted the importance of luminal bacteria to the immune dysregulation that is observed in Crohn's disease [8]. At this point, our working hypothesis incorporates the microbiome and immune dysregulation and is that Crohn's disease is caused by an abnormal immune response to luminal bacteria in a genetically susceptible host [1, 2].

1.2 Symptoms and Diagnosis

Patient symptoms often reflect the disease location. For example, patients with classic terminal ileal Crohn's disease can initially present with abdominal pain and may have minimal, if any, diarrhea. In these cases, first presentation may suggest irritable bowel syndrome (IBS) rather than the more serious diagnosis, IBD. Patients with predominately colonic Crohn's disease may have symptoms that are identical to other types of colitis resulting from infections, medications, or other causes and expressing symptoms of diarrhea, bloody stools, and urgency. Patients with disease in the stomach or upper small intestine may have serious dyspepsia mimicking peptic ulcer disease. For patients presenting with pain and diarrhea, the severity of symptoms along with "red flag" signs and symptoms such as blood in the stool, weight loss, anemia, and fever and high inflammatory markers including C-reactive protein (CRP) leads the clinician to suspect IBD. The onset of symptoms in the second or third decade of life or a family history of IBD adds to the suspicion [1]. Extraintestinal manifestations of IBD are immunologically driven and include spondylarthritis, erythema nodosum, pyoderma gangrenosum, primary sclerosing cholangitis, and uveitis; the presence or history of these conditions also suggests the diagnosis of IBD [9]. Finally, the presence of a perianal fistula or fistula to a scar, the body wall, bladder, or vagina, even historically, strongly suggests Crohn's disease and strongly favors Crohn's disease over ulcerative colitis in those cases where IBD is likely but the type of IBD is uncertain [1, 2].

Crohn's disease remains a disease where the diagnosis is made by a combination of patient history, suggestive laboratory features, and findings on imaging and histology, with no single diagnostic criteria confirmatory. Commonly obtained blood tests such as CRP can be supportive, is neither sensitive nor specific enough to be definitive. Tests that are more specific for gut inflammation include fecal calprotectin or lactoferrin. These tests are also supportive rather than diagnostic and are most sensitive for colonic inflammation. They are most commonly used once the disease is established to determine if ongoing or worsening symptoms are indicative of active inflammation and are used as a surrogate to avoid repeated invasive or expensive testing [1, 10].

1.3 Imaging the Bowel

Imaging, either cross-sectional imaging or endoscopic imaging, has become the standard for initial diagnosis, for evaluating Crohn's disease location and severity, and for assessing for complications [11]. When the diagnosis is new or uncertain, the initial test of choice for adult patients is generally colonoscopy as it is able to directly visualize the involvement and is able to obtain biopsies from the distal ileum and the colon for histologic analysis. The combination of typical endoscopic appearance and histologic findings of inflammation with evidence of chronicity, in the appropriate clinical setting, is the most reassuring to the caregiver that the diagnosis of Crohn's disease is convincingly made. Cross-sectional imaging is typically performed even when the new diagnosis of Crohn's disease seems secure, to examine the intestine proximal to the reach of the colonoscopy. When the diagnosis is less certain, noninvasive imaging such as CTE or MRE is frequently ordered if colonoscopy is negative and the index of suspicion remains high. For the new diagnosis of Crohn's disease, standard of care is such that most patients have both a colonoscopy and cross-sectional imaging for a complete evaluation of the GI tract. For patients with known disease, whether colonoscopy or cross- sectional imaging is requested depends on the patient's prior disease location, symptoms, prior imaging, and the questions to be asked. CTE or MRE is particularly useful when evaluating for complications of stricture, abscess, fistula, or obstruction. In patients who are too sick to take the colonoscopy preparation or when the procedure itself is risky, enterography becomes the best and sometimes only option for decision-making. From the GI perspective, the choice between CTE and MRE is often made by scan availability, patient tolerance, local radiologic expertise, and cost. In IBD centers in recent years, MRI use has eclipsed CT utilization due to added insights provided by the multiphasic MRI sequences and improved MRI availability and expertise [12].

Gastroenterologists have heard the message that CTE and MRE are the cross-sectional imaging modalities of choice for imaging the small intestine. Other radiographic modalities such as small bowel follow-through are largely of historical interest and cannot match the information derived from CTE and MRE. Capsule endoscopy is available at most centers and has some value when the index of suspicion is high and other testing is unrevealing. It appears that capsule endoscopy is the most sensitive method for assessing the small bowel [13, 14]. There are times when identifying subtle small bowel lesions will lend insight into patient symptoms when other imaging is negative, but most often, since therapeutics are generally not targeted, the exact localization of subtle lesions does not change medical management. In addition, unrecognized strictures can result in capsule retention which can require surgery. The often used argument that the surgery was inevitable does not seem patient centric and is not justified in most cases [14]. Ultrasound is promising and may be our best test for assessing tissue fibrosis, though it is highly operator dependent and not easily reproducible [15].

1.4 Imaging in the Biologic Era

The introduction of infliximab in the 1990s ushered in a new era of therapeutics. Hope was renewed that biologics, typified by infliximab, could alter the natural history of Crohn's disease. This is a concept that was all but abandoned with our prior classes of drugs including steroids, mesalamine, and their relatives. In 2018, the goal of altering the natural history of the disease and preventing the complications of stricture and fistula formation has not been completely realized. Hospitalization and surgical intervention rates are lower in many studies of patients on potent biologics, but the fibrosis seems to march on in many cases [4]. In addition, cost, side effects, and worry about long-term complications of the drugs can affect patient acceptance and cause physicians to switch from therapy to therapy. Surgery remains

Table 1.1 Therapeutic options in IBD

Medication type	Example
Mesalamine	Pentasa™, Asacol™, Lialda™
Steroid	Prednisone, Entocort™, Uceris™
Immunomodulator	Azathioprine, Methotrexate
Biologic	
Anti-TNFα	Infliximab (Remicade™), Adalimumab (Humira™), Certolizumab (Cimzia™)
Anti-integrin	Vedolizumab (Entyvio™)
Anti-IL12/IL23	Ustekinumab (Stelara™)
Small molecule	
JAK Inhibitor	Tofacitinib (Xeljanz™)

a reality for many patients, and recurrence rates of Crohn's disease postoperatively remain high [16]. It is clear that even given our promising new therapies, the disease is a challenge for physicians and patients and remains without a cure.

Our armamentarium has greatly expanded in the past two decades, and now we routinely use up to a dozen biologics and immunomodulators for modern IBD care (Table 1.1). The approach to therapeutics has also changed with a more aggressive approach using a "treat-to-target" philosophy. The most relevant target used in practice is mucosal healing [12]. Generally, this is based on colonoscopic healing, though using improved signs of inflammation on cross-sectional imaging as a therapeutic target is possible. Indeed, the data show that MRI may be more impactful than colonoscopy in determining patients' management [17]. A comprehensive system that incorporates structural information from several imaging sources is optimal [18]. The care of IBD patients has become multispecialty with radiologists playing an important role. While the care of IBD patients has become more complex, the questions that clinicians need answered to make informed decisions remain the same: where in the gut is the inflammation located, how severe is it, and are there any complications such as stricture, fistula, or abscess? A common and somewhat tougher question is whether sites of involvement and severity are consistent with the patient's symptoms. As technology improves and new data emerges, we are able to ask more sophisticated questions such as how is the current therapy working and what does the future hold for this patient? Noninvasive cross-sectional imaging holds promise to address many of the burning clinical questions that are critical to patient care.

1.5 Communicating with Gastroenterologists

There is no substitute for face-to-face interactions between radiologists and gastroenterologists to review scans and discuss particularly difficult cases. While this type of interaction may represent a bygone era, it remains the basis for a good working relationship. In the current practice environment where in-person interactions are less common, it is especially important that the imaging study report communicates the key and complete information about the scan along with comparison to past imaging. When coupled with the responsibility for identifying abnormal findings outside the gut and the pressures of case volume, this seems like an overwhelming task for our radiologists. From the gastroenterologists' perspective, the electronic medical record and the wide availability of computers have enhanced our ability to view scans in the clinic or the bedside and even demonstrate the findings to our patients. The opportunity to view primary data provides caregivers insights into disease processes that were previously only understood by surgeons in the operating room. When caregivers take time to review the scan with the patient, it boosts the patient's confidence in the process and enhances the patient's understanding of the need for potentially toxic medications. This leads to improved medication adherence and, ultimately, better control of disease symptoms.

Concern has been raised about the number of scans our Crohn's disease patients undergo in a disease lifetime. This was especially true during the early implementation of CT enterography when radiation dosages were high. Cumulative exposure remains a concern even for the low radiation procedures. Procedural issues related to patient anxiety, intolerance of oral and intravenous contrast, procedure cost, and respect for patient time remain the reasons to avoid overtesting. Overtesting can be the result of frequent emergency room visits or hospitalizations. Careful consideration can decrease overtesting in these cases. For example, only marginal added value is derived from a CT or MR enterography ordered immediately after a standard CT abdomen/pelvis performed in an emergency department [19]. In these cases, the images should be assessed and individualized for specific patient circumstances. This is where good communication between the radiologist and caregivers along with a careful detailed report will help educate caregivers and limit excessive use of cross-sectional imaging.

Effective communication is key when reporting disease activity. This is particularly important in reporting relative contributions of inflammation and fibrosis to an involved segment of bowel. Certain findings on CTE and MRE such as enhancement and mural stratification correlate extremely well with histologic and endoscopic inflammation [20–22]. Findings that reflect tissue fibrosis are less reliable. It is often assumed that an involved (thickened) segment without radiographic signs of inflammation is fibrotic. However, it seems that inflammation and fibrosis are closely pathologically linked such that even segments that lack radiographic signs of inflammation are histologically inflamed and the best marker of histologic fibrosis is inflammation [21]. Disease segments termed "inactive" or "fibrotic" or "chronic" can be misleading to caregivers and patients leading patients to question the need for continued medical therapy. This issue was addressed in the recent published joint consensus statement by the Society of Abdominal Radiology and the American Gastroenterological Association [23] and is an area where effective communication of findings is critical to medical decision-making.

Given that we are rarely given the privilege of time or proximity to have meaningful face-to-face interaction, most of the communication occurs through the order placed by the caregiver and the radiology report. Unfortunately, the order often contains generic requests such as "assess disease activity and evaluate for complications." This provides minimal information and guidance to the radiologist. Further, no standardized reporting rubric for CTE or MRE findings exists for CD as it does in reporting for other diseases. In a retrospective study of CTE and MRE reporting of radiographic exams in the electronic medical record, we found that findings of inflammation and serious complication such as fistula and abscess were communicated consistently but that findings suggesting bowel fibrosis such as stricture formation were often unreported [24]. This is an important issue since the finding of a fixed stricture predicts poor patient outcomes [25]. Therefore, it is important to communicate this information to the clinician so that this finding can be considered when formulating a treatment plan.

1.6 Wish List for Future Applications

Scope technology and the performance of colonoscopy have changed only incrementally in the last two decades. By contrast, CT and MR imaging have had paradigm-changing advances in safety, resolution, and the ability to distinguish normal and pathologic tissue layers. These advances, along with increased availability and expertise, have allowed the use of CT and MR enterography to ask new questions about disease management. We now know that MRE is sensitive to changes in inflammation that occur with biologic therapy allowing the use of MRE as a biomarker in clinical trials of new therapies [26]. We also know that findings of enterography can be used to predict disease outcomes, forcing us all to think beyond the static findings at a single point in time [25, 27]. It is anticipated that the ability to predict disease course will be the imaging frontier for care of IBD patients. To make this possible, new sequences aimed at better characterizing of tissue fibrosis, the pathologic consequence of inflammation that leads to complications such as stricture and fistula formation, are needed. The relative contribution of inflammation vs. fibrosis in an involved segment is clinically important as it informs the decision as to medical vs. surgical therapy. MRI sequences such as the cine sequences [28] and magnetization transfer [29] are being explored for better assessment of tissue fibrosis and are evidence of the increased power of MRI over CT for providing disease-relevant information beyond location and severity of inflammation. Co-registration of voxels over time in a single exam to account for bowel motion, and between exams to assess disease course, is a new horizon. Using registration to combine different modalities has potential in the gut as it does in the brain and the heart. The future offers endless possibilities for this powerful technology. The full potential can be realized when clinicians, radiologists, and MR physicists work together to solve burning clinical problems.

1.7 Conclusion

Cross-sectional imaging in Crohn's disease has greatly improved our understanding of the pathophysiology of the disease. It has a proven role in diagnosing Crohn's disease, in assessing symptoms, and in identifying disease complications. Emerging data support the ability of cross- sectional imaging to predict future disease complications. Modern care of patients with Crohn's disease requires a multidisciplinary team approach. Cross talk between gastroenterologists and radiologists has resulted in improved interpretation and reporting and expanded utilization of imaging findings in patient care. Cross-sectional imaging impacts modern Crohn's disease management strategies in profound ways, and radiologists have a critical role on the multidisciplinary care team.

References

1. Ananthakrishan AN, Xavier RJ, Podolsky DK. Inflammatory bowel disease: pathogenesis. In: Podolsky DK, et al., editors. Yamada's textbook of gastroenterology. 6th ed. New York: Wiley; 2016. p. 1364–77.
2. Torres J, Mehandru S, Colombel JF, Peyrin-Biroulet L. Crohn's disease. Lancet. 2017;389:1741–55.
3. Cosnes J, Gower-Rousseau C, Seksik P, Cortot A. Epidemiology and natural history of inflammatory bowel diseases. Gastroenterology. 2011;140:1785–94.
4. Latella R, Sferra R, Speca S, Vetuschi A, Gaudio E. Can we prevent, reduce or reverse intestinal fibrosis in IBD? Eur Rev Med Pharmacol Sci. 2013;17:1283–304.
5. Khor B, Gardet A, Xavier RJ. Genetics and pathogenesis of inflammatory bowel disease. Nature. 2011;474:307–17.
6. Li Q, Lee CH, Peters LA, Mastropaolo LA, Thoeni C, Elkadri A, Schwerd T, Zhu J, Zhang B, Zhao Y, Hao K, Dinarzo A, Hoffman G, Kidd BA, Murchie R, Al Adham Z, Guo C, Kotlarz D, Cutz E, Walters TD, Shouval DS, Curran M, Dobrin R, Brodmerkel C, Snapper SB, Klein C, Brumell JH, Hu M, Nanan R, Snanter-Nanan B, Wong M, Le Deist F, Haddad E, Roifman CM, Deslandres C, Griffiths AM, Gaskin KJ, Uhlig HH, Schadt EE, Muise AM. Variants in TRIM22 that affect NOD2 Signaling are associated with very-early-onset inflammatory bowel disease. Gastroenterology. 2016;150:1196–207.
7. Al Nabhani Z, Dietrich G, Hugot JP, Barreau F. Nod2: the intestinal gate keeper. PLoS Pathog. 2017;13:e1006177. https://doi.org/10.1371/journal.ppat.1006177.
8. de Souza HSP, Fiocchi C, Iliopoulos D. The IBD interactome: an integrated view of aetiology, pathogenesis and therapy. Nat Rev Gastroenterol Hepatol. 2017;14:739–49.
9. Isene R, Bernklev T, Høie O, Munkholm P, Tsianos E, Stockbrügger R, Odes S, Palm O, Småstuen M, Moum B, The Ec-Ibd Study Group. Extraintestinal manifestations in Crohn's disease and ulcerative colitis: results from a prospective, population-based European inception cohort. Scand J Gastroenterol. 2015;50:300–5.
10. Ministro P, Martins D. Fecal biomarkers in inflammatory bowel disease: how, when and why? Expert Rev Gastroenterol Hepatol. 2017;11:317–28.
11. Bruining DH, Bhatnagar G, Rimola J, Taylor S, Zimmermann EM, Fletcher JG. CT and MR imaging in Crohn's disease: current and future applications. Abdom Imaging. 2015;40:965–74.
12. Colombel JF, Narula N, Peyrin-Biroulet L. Management strategies to improve outcomes of patients with inflammatory bowel diseases. Gastroenterology. 2017;152:351–61.
13. Enns RA, Hookey L, Armstrong D, Bernstein CN, Heitman SJ, Teshima C, Leontiadis GI, Tse F, Sadowski D. Clinical practice guidelines for the use of video capsule endoscopy. Gastroenterology. 2017;152:497–514.
14. Kopylov U, Ben-Horin S, Seidman EG, Eliakim R. Video capsule endoscopy of the small bowel for monitoring of Crohn's disease. Inflamm Bowel Dis. 2015;21:2726–35.
15. Quaia E, Gennari AG, Cova MA, van Beek EJR. Differentiation of inflammatory from fibrotic ileal strictures among patients with Crohn's disease based on visual analysis: feasibility study combining conventional B-mode ultrasound, contrast-enhanced ultrasound and strain elastography. Ultrasound Med Biol. 2018;44:762–70.
16. Peyrin-Biroulet L, Harmsen WS, Tremaine WJ, et al. Surgery in a population-based cohort of Crohn's disease from Olmsted County, Minnesota (1970–2004). Am J Gastroenterol. 2012;107:1693–701.
17. Bosch OG, Ordâs I, Rodriguez S, et al. Comparison of the impact of MRI and colonoscopy on management of Crohn's disease. Gastroenterology. 2012;142:S-21–2.
18. Pariente B, Mary JY, Danese S, et al. Development of the Lémann index to assess digestive tract damage in patients with Crohn's disease. Gastroenterology. 2015;148:52–63.
19. Schreyer AG, Hoffstetter P, Daneschnejad M, Jung EM, Pawlik M, Friedrich C, Fellner C, Strauch U, Klebl F, Herfarth H, Zorger N. Comparison of conventional abdominal CT with MR-enterography in patients with active Crohn's disease and acute abdominal pain. Acad Radiol. 2010;17:352–7.

20. Rimola J, Planell N, Rodríguez S, Delgado S, Ordás I, Ramírez-Morros A, et al. Characterization of inflammation and fibrosis in Crohn's disease lesions by magnetic resonance imaging. Am J Gastroenterol. 2015;110:432–40.
21. Adler J, Punglia D, Dillman JR, Polydorides AD, Dave M, Al-Hawary MM, Platt JF, McKenna GJ, Zimmermann EM. CT enterography findings correlate with tissue inflammation in resected small bowel Crohn's disease. Inflamm Bowel Dis. 2012;18:849–56.
22. Wagner M, Ko HM, Chatterji M, Besa C, Torres J, Zhang X, Panchal H, Hectors S, Cho J, Colombel JF, Harpaz N, Taouli B. Magnetic resonance imaging predicts histopathologic composition of ileal Crohn's disease. J Crohns Colitis. 2018;12(6):718–29.
23. Bruining DH, Zimmermann EM, Loftus EV, Sanborn WJ, Sauer CG, Strong SA. Consensus guidelines for evaluation, interpretation and utilization of CT and MR enterography in small bowel Crohn's disease patients. Radiology. 2018;286(3):776–99.
24. Flint A, Chaudhry NA, Riverso M, Pham, A, Moser PP, Mramba LK, Zimmermann EM, Grajo JR. Effective communication of cross-sectional imaging findings in Crohn's disease: comparing conventional EMR reporting to a published scoring system. Abdom Radiol. 2017. https://doi.org/10.1007/s00261-017-1368-0.
25. Chaudhry NA, Riverso M, Grajo JR, Moser PP, Zou F, Homsi M, Punglia DR, Zimmermann EM. A fixed stricture on routine cross sectional imaging predicts disease-related complications and adverse outcomes in patients with Crohn's disease. Inflamm Bowel Dis. 2017;23:641–9.
26. Castiglione F, Mainenti P, Testa A, Imperatore N, De Palma GD, Maurea S, Rea M, Nardone OM, Sanges M, Caporaso N, Rispo A. Cross-sectional evaluation of transmural healing in patients with Crohn's disease on maintenance treatment with anti-TNF alpha agents. Dig Liver Dis. 2017;49:484–9.
27. Fiorino G, Peyrin-Biroulet L, Bonifacio C, et al. MRE and colonoscopy findings in early Crohn's disease predict the course of the disease: a prospective observational cohort study. Gastroenterology. 2013;144:S-639.
28. Bickelhaupt S, Pazahr S, Chuck N, Blume I, Froehlich JM, Cattin R, Raible S, Bouquet H, Bill U, Rogler G, Frei P, Boss A, Patak MA. Crohn's disease: small bowel motility impairment correlates with inflammatory-related markers C-reactive protein and calprotectin. Neurogastroenterol Motil. 2013;25:467–73.
29. Li XH, Mao R, Huang SY, Sun CH, Cao QH, Fang ZN, Zhang ZW, Huang L, Lin JJ, Chen YJ, Rimola J, Rieder F, Chen MH, Feng ST, Li ZP. Characterization of degree of intestinal fibrosis in patients with Crohn disease by using magnetization transfer MR imaging. Radiology. 2018;287:494–503.

Bowel Ultrasound Imaging, Protocol and Findings

2

Astrid-Jane Greenup and Kerri L. Novak

Abstract

Objective measurement of disease activity in inflammatory bowel disease (IBD) is important to guide targeted therapy. Noninvasive approaches are gaining clinical traction given patient preference and need for cost containment. Ultrasound of the large and small bowel is increasingly recognized as an accurate, non-radiation-based, cost-effective modality useful in both diagnosis and follow-up in IBD. Intestinal ultrasound (IUS) is easily repeated, allowing for serial assessment to evaluate response to therapy, post-operative course and evolution of complications, particularly in Crohn's disease. Mounting evidence suggesting sonographic response accurately reflects therapeutic efficacy and thus may provide useful insight regarding clinical outcome. It exhibits similar performance in the detection of inflammation associated with Crohn's disease to both computed tomography (CT) and magnetic resonance (MR). Intestinal US may also provide a noninvasive surrogate to ileocolonoscopy, accurately depicting disease activity and mucosal healing, with better illustration of luminal and extra-luminal disease and complications. Intestinal US may also play a role in depicting the activity, extent of disease as well as risk of surgery in ulcerative colitis. The application of IUS is particularly useful in children with IBD, where risks of radiation are important, while there is a need for anaesthesia for endoscopic examination. To date, however, IUS has remained somewhat underutilized globally, given perceived limitations in inter-rater variability, standardized assessment and anatomic resolution. This however is starting to change: the use of IUS has moved beyond the limited domain of diagnostic imaging specialists and radiologists as it is incorporated into routine clinical assessment at the bedside and now being

A.-J. Greenup
Liverpool Hospital, University of New South Wales, Sydney, NSW, Australia

K. L. Novak (✉)
University of Calgary, Calgary, AB, Canada
e-mail: knovak@ucalgary.ca

J. Rimola (ed.), *Cross-Sectional Imaging in Crohn's Disease*,
https://doi.org/10.1007/978-3-319-96586-4_2

performed by non-radiologist gastroenterologists. Here, the benefits to patients go well beyond safety, with immediate clinical impact, facilitated through objectively informed clinical decision-making and better patient education and engagement, allowing for optimal patient participation and partnership in the clinical management of this complex, chronic disease.

2.1 Introduction

Intestinal ultrasound (IUS) is a useful alternate to existing modalities available for luminal and cross-sectional evaluation of the small and large bowel in inflammatory bowel disease (IBD) since it was first used in Crohn's disease (CD) just over 35 years ago [1]. Imaging is fundamental to evaluation at the outset as part of diagnosis and in the follow-up of IBD [2]. Objective markers of disease have become part of standard monitoring algorithms, given recognized disconnect between disease activity and symptoms [3, 4]. However, patient preference, safety and cost are increasingly recognized as important drivers in monitoring choice, with noninvasive options given priority. Therefore, the application of IUS in IBD is gaining momentum, with an expanding array of indications, ranging from diagnosis and assessment of early response to therapy to post-operative surveillance and assessment of perianal disease in CD. Enhanced image resolution related to improving technology, including use of higher-frequency probes, harmonic imaging and better imaging of low blood flow vasculature with colour Doppler, further enables wider adoption.

Although extant evidence suggests IUS accuracy rivals either traditional imaging modality, namely, computed tomography with enterography (CT/CTE) and magnetic resonance enterography (MRE), IUS has remained underutilized [5]. Similar to MRE, a salient benefit of IUS is safety, given the absence of ionizing radiation, useful even during pregnancy. Preparation is also minimal, while the significant value of IUS also uniquely rests in the capacity to perform an assessment while engaging the patient directly, unlike with CT or MR. This patient interaction with IUS enables education and empowerment regarding findings of disease activity, inactivity and stability, with opportunity for explication for the continuation, commencement or cessation of potentially impactful, costly medical therapy.

In addition to the advantages related to patient tolerance and engagement, IUS can provide information beyond that generated from more traditional methods of disease assessment. From a technical viewpoint, IUS is unique in the real-time ability to assess bowel function concurrently with structure. Unlike endoscopic assessment, assessment for transmural complications, such as the development of fistulas or abscesses, can occur concurrently with that of luminal disease activity. Accompanying techniques to standard IUS such as contrast enhancement and elastography show promise for improved, safe characterization of fibrosis and complications. Such techniques include the use of contrast, via oral or intravenous (IV) administration, as well as the use of elastography. The latter will be explored in further detail in subsequent chapters (Chaps. 4 and 8).

The use of both basic IUS in addition to the aforementioned techniques have enabled consideration of the development of objective scoring systems for disease activity, mirroring similar endeavours in endoscopic and other imaging fields (Chap. 10). Incorporation of such scoring systems into standardized IUS reports will further contribute to reproducibility, minimization of observer variation and the ability to accurately monitor disease progression with IUS, all of which are desired features of any disease activity assessment tool in CD, particularly in the era of treat to target. Despite the many strengths of IUS in the assessment of CD, potential limitations demand discussion. This chapter will outline existing evidence supporting the accuracy of IUS, its contribution in the assessment of IBD as well as summarizing the technical aspects of performing and reporting IUS.

2.2 Intestinal Ultrasound Compared to Other Modalities for the Diagnosis and Monitoring of Inflammatory Bowel Disease

With the developing momentum of US in the field of CD, parameters of activity have been studied individually and in combination, to assess correlation with other indicators of disease activity. Adjunctive techniques to standard IUS can enhance accuracy, including the use of contrast, both oral and intravenous administration, as well as the use of elastography (explored in further detail in Chaps. 4 and 8).

2.2.1 Crohn's Disease

2.2.1.1 Diagnosis of Crohn's Disease

Intestinal US has consistently demonstrated comparable accuracy to other imaging modalities such as CTE and MRE for the diagnosis of CD, with a sensitivity and specificity ranging between 75 and 100% [5, 6]. Diagnosis is based largely on bowel wall thickness [7]. Intestinal US has documented superior diagnostic capacity for disease located in the ileum and sigmoid and descending colon and more so when compared to that located in the rectum, duodenum and proximal jejunum [7–9]. Similarly, IUS consistently accurately identifies disease activity in the context of established disease, when compared to endoscopy or alternate cross-sectional imaging [7]. Similar to alternate imaging modalities, the accuracy of IUS for the assessment of the extent of disease does vary in the reported literature. Small intestinal contrast enhancement, through ingestion of oral iso-osmolar contrast, has been reported to increase the accuracy of IUS, with reported improved detection of proximal small bowel lesions, complications and extent of disease [7, 10].

2.2.1.2 Response to Therapy

Historically, endpoints in both clinical trials and clinical practice focused principally on the reporting of symptoms by patients; however, it is well recognized such measures are inadequate in accurately reflecting disease activity [11]. Accordingly, therapeutic targets have evolved beyond symptomatic remission to include measures of mucosal healing. Currently, ileocolonoscopy is the gold standard for assessment of mucosal healing; however, it is not amendable to serial evaluation, nor is it able to assess transmural healing. Alternatively, IUS can be repeated in short intervals allowing for early and frequent monitoring of therapeutic response, with the important benefit of being well tolerated. Additionally, IUS can accurately assess transmural inflammation, as an excellent surrogate for endoscopic healing with high correlation in the terminal ileum and in the colon [12]. Longer-term follow-up by both IUS and MR similarly demonstrates complete transmural healing in those with moderate to severe CD, less than may be expected based on symptom profile and clinical remission rates [13–15]. The significance of transmural healing and its role in predicting outcome however is not yet completely understood.

Early detection of non-response or loss of response to therapy may allow for optimal therapeutic management and enhanced long-term outcomes. In paediatrics, response to antitumour necrosis factor (anti-TNF) occurs as early as 2 weeks, with close correlation to faecal calprotectin (fCP) [16]. Moreover, demonstration of early response to therapy with IUS has been shown to predict response on IUS at 12 months and improve outcome [13, 17]. Radiologic response is an important predictor of outcome: even partial response as seen on cross-sectional imaging is associated with improved long-term outcomes such as need for corticosteroids, surgery and hospitalization [18].

2.2.1.3 Detection of Complications

Intestinal US is accurate in the detection of IBD-related complications such as strictures, enteric fistulae and abscesses. In multiple studies, IUS has a pooled sensitivity for detecting strictures of 79% (95% CI 71–84%) and specificity of 92% (95% CI 87–96%) when compared to surgical specimens. Intestinal US has a comparable accuracy to CT and MR for the detection of strictures [19]. Assessment of the degree of inflammation or fibrosis in strictures can be enhanced with the addition of contrast, enabling an important differentiation when therapeutic decisions are being made. Similarly, IUS has a pooled sensitivity for detecting enteric fistulae of 74% (95% CI 67–79%) and specificity of 95% (95% CI 91–97%) when compared to surgical specimens, while the addition of contrast can be used to assess fistula tracts. Intestinal US has a pooled sensitivity for detecting abscesses of 84% and a specificity of 93% when compared to surgery. Furthermore, contrast enhanced US, although extant data is limited, has been shown to be highly accurate (accuracy of 97.2%) when compared to either alternate imaging or gross pathology in the differentiation of inflammatory phlegmons from intra-abdominal abscesses [20]. Additionally, IUS is able to assess structural bowel damage with accuracy comparable to MRE. In CD, bowel damage can be quantified using the sonographic lesion index for Crohn's disease (SLIC) [21].

2.2.1.4 Evaluation of Post-Operative Recurrence

Traditional methods of monitoring patients post-operatively include symptoms, serologic measurement of C-reactive protein (CRP), fCP and endoscopic activity. Intestinal US can provide a greater depth of information, including the extent of disease or presence of post-operative complications with equal or greater accuracy when compared to these methods [22]. While ileocolonoscopy remains the gold standard for post-operative monitoring, IUS has also been shown to be an accurate modality for diagnosing post-operative recurrence, with post-operative IUS findings being closely correlated to findings from ileocolonoscopy [22–24] (Fig. 2.1). Intestinal US is also useful for serial monitoring for recurrence of disease in patients who have undergone

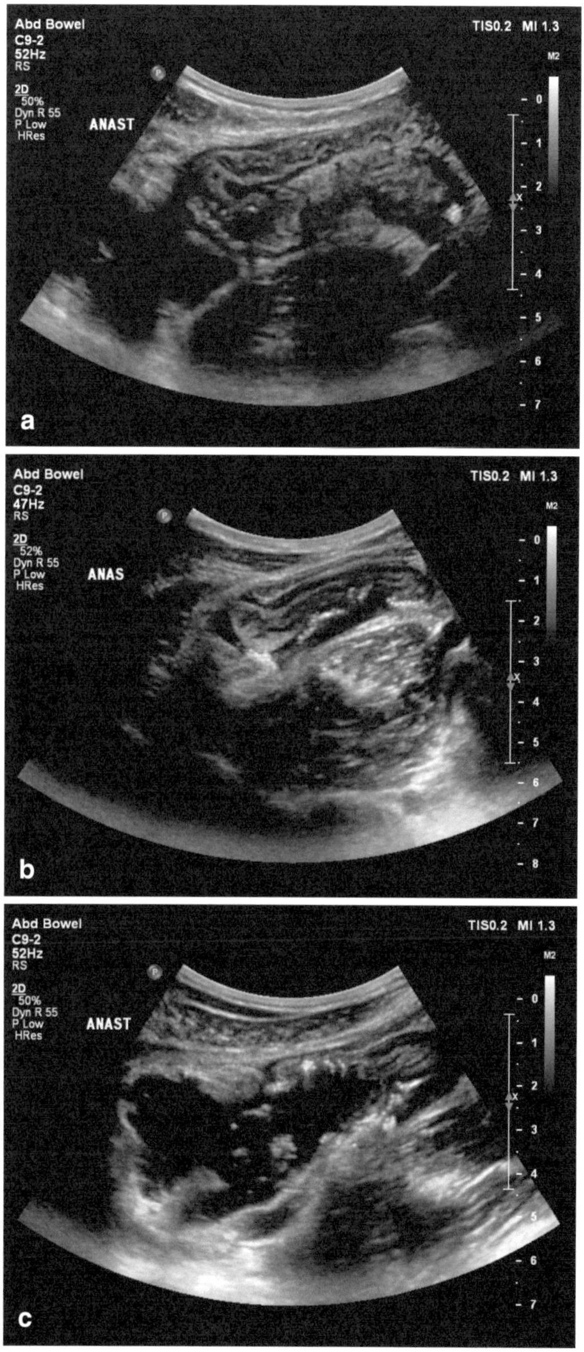

Fig. 2.1 This image depicts a 76 year old man, with emergent ileocolic resection 6 months prior, with ongoing significant diarrhoea and recurrence of the ileal side of the anastomosis. (**a**) Demonstrates the neoterminal ileum, emanating off of the side-to-side anastomosis on the superior margin. In (**b**), the blind end of the ileal side of the side-to-side anastomosis, with regular hyperechoic staples seen on the border with the fluid-filled colon. In (**c**), the colon is fluid filled, with staples seen on the medial side, joining the blind-ended ileum

intestinal resection, with the benefit of negating the need for multiple endoscopies. Future studies are needed to correlate fCP and IUS in the post-operative period, which may further increase the sensitivity of fCP for even more effective noninvasive detection of recurrence.

2.2.1.5 Evaluation of Perianal Disease

Pelvic MRI is the gold standard test for imaging perianal CD, but cost and availability may limit accessibility for assessment, particularly when urgent drainage is the primary concern. Transperineal US is a viable alternative that is accurate compared to MRI in the detection for both perianal lesions and complications such as fistulae and abscesses (see Chap. 9), readily available and easily repeated during the clinical assessment [25, 26].

2.2.1.6 Intestinal Ultrasound in Paediatrics

The prevalence of paediatric-onset IBD is increasing [27]. Objective monitoring of disease activity is particularly important to avoid the negative impact on growth and development. Computed tomography should be avoided if possible, given increased potential detriment from radiation exposure [28]. Monitoring with endoscopy is limited given the need for anaesthesia; in addition, young children often require anaesthesia for MRE, a modality with lengthy acquisition time, potentially lying prone while requiring breath holding, which is challenging for young children. Similar to adults, dedicated small bowel imaging is recommended for all children at diagnosis of IBD, in addition to ileocolonoscopy [29]. Magnetic resonance imaging is considered gold standard for imaging children with IBD, with the above noted limitation; thus not surprisingly, the use of IUS within the paediatric population is gaining momentum [30]. Intestinal US has been demonstrated to have a similar sensitivity and specificity as MRI when both were compared with the endoscopy for the diagnosis of IBD in paediatric patients for whom there was clinical suspicion; however, support from additional well-designed US trials to demonstrate utility is important [31]. Bowel wall thickness and complications (stricture, fistulae, abscesses) exhibit the greatest agreement when comparing readers. Early sonographic response in paediatrics including reduction in the length of disease, bowel wall thickness, mesenteric fat and colour Doppler signal of the wall and mesentery in response to anti-TNF therapy has been documented as early as 2 weeks [16]. Demonstration of a strong correlation of IUS activity with fCP following therapy was also documented [16]. Nonetheless, given potential limitations with IUS in detection of rectal and proximal small disease, it is recommended by the ESPGHAN revised Porto criteria for the diagnosis of IBD in children that in the preliminary diagnostic workup of paediatric patients with suspected IBD, IUS should be complemented by more sensitive imaging of the small bowel such as MRE [29, 32].

2.2.2 Ultrasound in Ulcerative Colitis

Given the safety, tolerability and opportunity for accessible serial monitoring in CD, the applicability of IUS has also been considered in ulcerative colitis (UC). One may assume IUS to be inadequate given pathological changes of UC characteristically being limited to the mucosa; however, on the contrary, IUS has been shown to have reasonable capacity to provide information surrounding both the degree of active and chronic inflammation in the left and right colon. This is of particular importance in attempts to distinguish UC from CD and indeterminate colitis [33, 34]. It is acknowledged however that consistent, satisfactory rectal viewing is limited.

The primary role of endoscopic assessment in establishing the initial diagnosis of UC is established; however, IUS could be of benefit in scenarios where endoscopic evaluation is not possible, including the potential for establishing disease extent beyond the rectum in acute severe UC. Another useful role for IUS is for monitoring of disease activity and assessment of response to therapy. It may also contribute to characterizing some of the chronic changes associated with poorly controlled, fibrotic disease including loss of haustra and the increased hyperechoic submucosal layer (the "lead pipe" endoscopic appearance), with decreased intramural vascularity as seen with Doppler [35, 36]. Intestinal US exhibits high concordance (weighted kappa between 0.76 and 0.9) between repetitive endoscopic and sonographic assessments when reported in 74 patients with UC over a 15-month period [37]. Furthermore, it may be predictive: both endoscopic and IUS scores at 3 months were found to be associated with a high likelihood of endoscopic activity at 15 months. Intestinal US is a complement to endoscopic assessment in UC, adding value given the ease of this cross-sectional imaging addition (Fig. 2.2).

2.2.3 Summary

Mounting evidence, easy repeatability and cost-effectiveness argue for increasing use of IUS to objectively evaluate the small and large bowel in IBD, for both children and adults. The greatest likely application of IUS is in follow-up, to characterize response to therapy and monitoring of complications as a complement to baseline MRE and endoscopy where possible. Where it can be applied in the clinic setting, IUS provides a tool to help clinicians make accurate decisions as well as engage patients and family members through demonstrations aimed to improve understanding of disease and facilitate optimal medical management.

2.3 Basic Ultrasound Principles and Intestinal Ultrasound Technique

2.3.1 Scanning Technique and Approach

Reflection of acoustic energy between interfaces is the underlying premise for all applications of US, including the bowel. The amplitude of such reflected energy is used to generate US images with increasing computational capacity. Acoustic energy is transmitted via a range of transducers differing in their arrays, including linear, curved, phased or annular arrays, and in their frequency. Linear transducers are arranged in a linear fashion, with a resultant rectangular image, while convex curves produce a pie-shaped image. Transducer selection is key to optimal imaging, largely dictated by the desired depth of penetration, where the highest US frequency

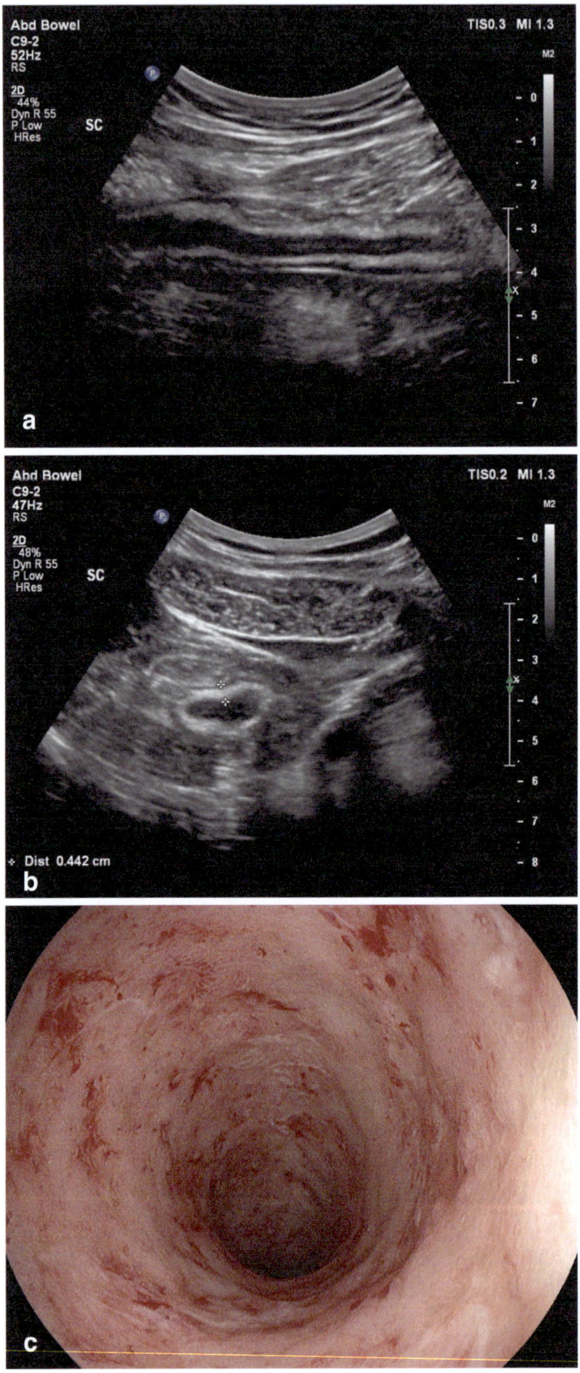

Fig. 2.2 A 28-year-old man diagnosed with extensive ulcerative colitis diagnosed in 2011 and lost to follow-up returns to care with increasing symptoms. In (**a**), note is made in the longitudinal image (oblique orientation) of the sigmoid colon, highlighting loss of normal folding and haustra, with increased echogenic submucosal layer (*thin arrow*). In (**b**), the same region, the sigmoid colon, in axial orientation documenting increased wall thickness, preservation of wall layers, and minimal surrounding mesenteric fat. In (**c**), flexible sigmoidoscopy was performed on the same day, confirming moderately severe (Mayo score 2) ulcerative colitis

is permitting minimal penetration but high resolution. For deeper structures, frequencies as low as 1.0–5.0 MHz may be required, commonly used in a general abdominal examination; more superficial structures like bowel are better visualized using imaging frequencies of 2.0–4.0 MHz to 12 MHz depending on the thickness of abdominal wall [38].

Before a comprehensive IUS assessment, review of all prior endoscopic, other cross-sectional imaging and IUS reports is helpful, particularly where prior surgery or known anatomical variation is relevant. With the patient in a supine position, an initial IUS assessment best comprises an initial overview of the abdomen using a transducer most suitable for the patient's body habitus. A low-frequency convex probe (1.0–5 MHz) is ideal for heavy patients, while a 2–4 to 9 MHz curved transducer is ideal for most patients. The deeper pelvic structures, including the rectum, are similarly best viewed with this lower-frequency probe. Further detailed characterization, once the anatomic location is well recognized, is ideally undertaken with a high-frequency linear array transducer (4–13 MHz), particularly where the abdominal wall is thin.

There is variability in the approach used amongst experts to assess the small and large bowel; however, for many, following a pathway mirroring assessment during colonoscopy is useful (distal to proximal). In such an instance, colonic examination can be initiated with the low-frequency probe being first placed over the rectum while using the bladder as an acoustic window, with images in both sagittal and transverse orientations. Following identification of the rectum, there is then a change to the higher-frequency probe (2–9 MHz). The large intestine is recognized by its haustra, larger size and relatively fixed location in the descending colon and hepatic flexure in the ascending colon. The sigmoid colon can then be identified and traced around to the descending colon, moving proximally to the transverse colon. The caecum is visualized as a blind-ending sac with an appendix if not resected and ileocecal valve. Ease of identifying the sigmoid colon is facilitated by delineating the psoas muscle and iliac vessels in the left lower quadrant, used as guide, with fanning cranially. It is important to note that the ascending and descending colon are generally located dorsolaterally on the right and left, respectively, whereas the transverse and sigmoid colon can have a more variable position due to its mesentery. Given the superior location of flexures, visualization of the hepatic and splenic flexures can be improved with inspiration and breath holding. Compression with the transducer and repositioning of the patient are integral components of identifying bowel as with standard US examinations. It is important to evaluate the medial and lateral aspects of the colon, to ensure characterization of extra-luminal features of disease. Consistent, standardized documentation of each section of the colon is important, including images in both sagittal/oblique, to ensure good longitudinal depiction, transverse and axial, as well as images with colour Doppler and bowel wall thickness measurement, clearly demarcating where in the abdomen the images were obtained.

An alternative approach is to begin the assessment in the right iliac fossa. Similarly, here the right psoas muscle and iliac vessels are landmarks used to identify the terminal ileum, which is generally the first bowel loop crossing from medial to lateral. The terminal ileum can be followed to the ileocecal valve and caecum; however, it can be deep emanating caudally from a low-lying caecum and ileocecal valve, important not to miss. The identification of the appendix, although challenging when normal, may also be possible often at the deep/caudal margin of the caecum, important to view in transverse and sagittal plane, with documentation of the blind end. It is usually 5–9 cm in length, arising from the dorsomedial wall of the caecum, a few centimetres from the ileocecal valve with variable orientation—retrocaecal, medial, anterior or posterior to the terminal ileum [39]. The ascending colon should be traced towards the hepatic flexure, with subsequent continuation along the transverse colon towards the descending, sigmoid colon and rectum.

The stomach wall with its rugae can be identified within the mid-epigastrium or left upper quadrant, often just lateral to the left lobe of the liver and requires differentiation from lower gastrointestinal structures (colon) by its three distinct layers on US [40].

The small bowel can be assessed commencing with the terminal ileum or neo-terminal ileum in post-operative state, subsequently tracing it as proximally as possible. Mapping of the small bowel in its entirety is difficult; therefore, ensuring a systematic approach is important, such as scanning the abdomen in parallel overlapping "lanes" [38]. Sweeps of the bowel and images of the bowel in long and short axis to ensure continuity are captured for review. The small bowel is characterized by valvulae conniventes when the lumen is fluid filled and active peristalsis that is not seen with the colon. Proximal small bowel tends to have longer conniventes; however, transition from jejunum to ileum is subjectively estimated with jejunal loops commonly present in the left upper quadrant.

Bowel preparation is considered optional, while prior fasting for 4–6 h may improve potential limitations associated by excessive bowel gas, although luminal air can provide contrast that may improve identification and characterization, such as colonic assessment, with a characteristic stool and air pattern (Fig. 2.3) [41]. It is also worth noting that the proximity to a recent meal will influence splanchnic blood flow, as will preceding physical activity. Contrary to protocols for CTE and MRE, the use of antispasmodics is not recommended in the performance of bowel ultrasound, and indeed the observation of motility is an important contributor to assess disease activity and altered motility associated with complications such as stricture [41].

The use of colour or power Doppler enables detection of blood flow which is best optimized to detect low flow within the smaller vessels of the intestinal wall [38]. Settings vary, but the lowest velocity scale combined with maximum sensitivity with avoidance of "noise" or artefact is ideal to isolate the signal to the surround mesentery and bowel wall. Colour Doppler signal then can provide a semi-qualitative measurement of active inflammation rated from 0 = no detection; 1 = very little flow, seen as fewer than two colour signals in a square centimetre; 2 = moderate; and 3= abundant flow within the region of interest [42]. Signals should persist within the wall or mesentery consistently, unlike movement artefact. There are a few possible explanations for a false-negative signal, including deep-lying loop or increased abdominal wall adiposity. If a high index of suspicion exists for activity, intravenous contrast enhancement may definitively clarify and quantify the presence of blood flow.

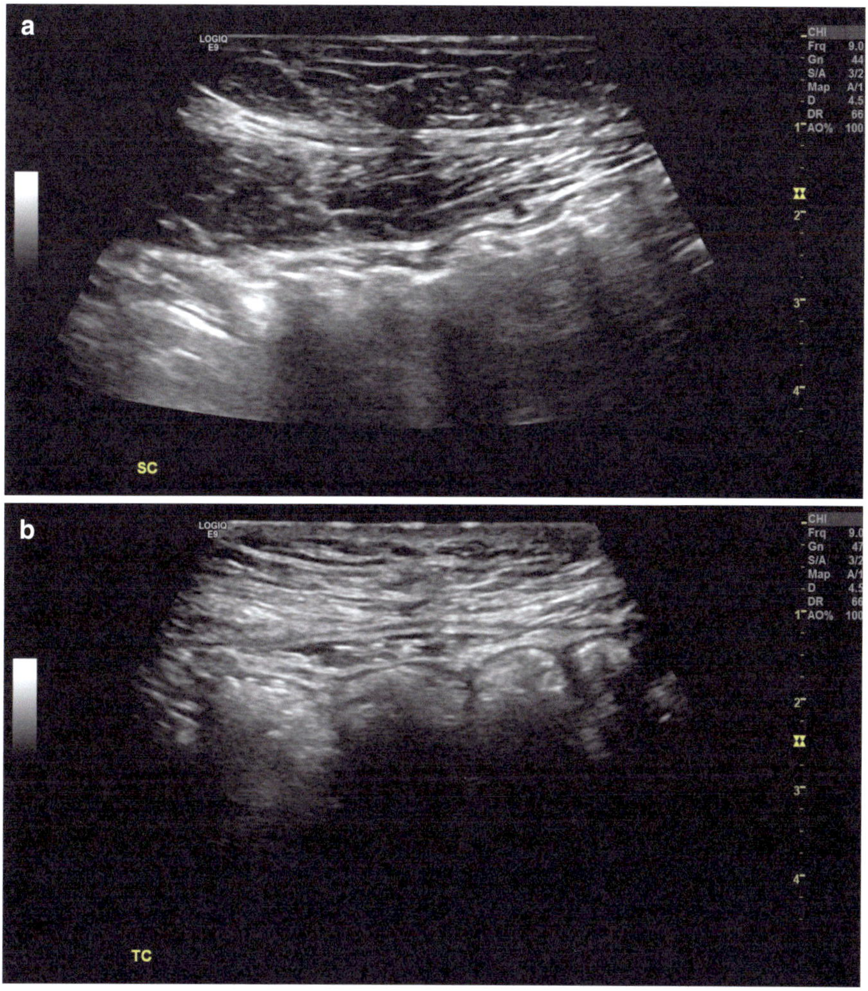

Fig. 2.3 Bowel evaluation beginning in the left lower quadrant, using curved 9–2 MHz probe, with longitudinal depiction of a normal sigmoid colon, characterized by thin (<2.0 mm) bowel wall and normal echostratification, with evidence of normal folds and haustra. The echogenic margin of the wall demonstrates air-containing stool. (**b**) Transverse image of the transverse colon, demonstrating normal haustral folds and stool pattern

2.4 Sonographic Features of Normal Bowel and Inflammatory Activity

The fundamental components to bowel assessment include the length of the affected bowel, wall thickness and echostratification (preservation/loss of normal layers), in addition to the assessment of surrounding mesenteric lymph nodes and fat (Fig. 2.4). Additional features of interest include findings suggestive of impending or present

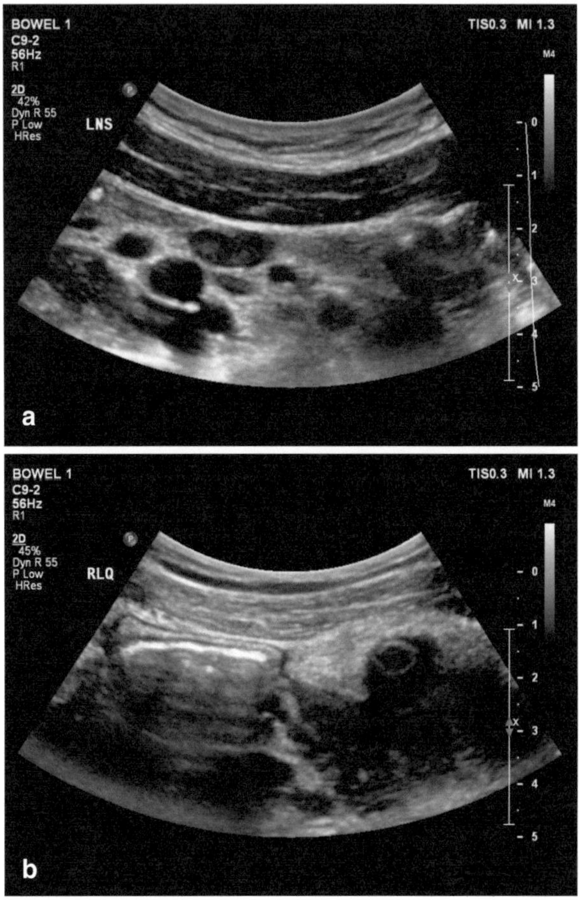

Fig. 2.4 A 33-year-old mother of two healthy children, with long-standing chronic ulcerative colitis on an anti-TNF biosimilar presented to clinic with severe abdominal pain, abdominal distention, and 2-week history of fever. She was found to have a perforated appendix. (**a**) Demonstrates abundant, large reactive lymph nodes in the right lower quadrant, while (**b**) highlights the "halo" of inflammatory fat (*arrow*) that surrounds the tip of the appendix that has a probably pus-filled collection on its inferior edge

perforation, namely, spiculation of the serosal aspect of the bowel wall, or that of abscess formation. Finally, as aforementioned, peristaltic activity provides further insight into the health of the examined bowel, best captured as video clips length 15–25 s.

2.4.1 Bowel Wall Stratification

Five layers of the bowel wall may be appreciated sonographically given alternating echogenic (bright) and hypoechoic (dark) characteristics of the corresponding histologic layers, moving in the luminal to serosal direction in alternating echogenic and hypoechoic layers: mucosa (Layer 1), hypoechoic muscularis mucosa (Layer 2), echogenic submucosa (Layer 3), hypoechoic muscularis propria (Layer 4) and serosa interface (Layer 5) (Fig. 2.5). Such a correlation differs slightly when focusing on the dorsal wall, while this aspect is not always easily visualized due to air in the lumen, and hence it is recommended that measurements are made in the anterior bowel wall [38]. For practical purposes, three layers are visualized consistently, Layers 2–4 (dark or hypoechoic, light/hyperechoic and then dark). Loss of bowel

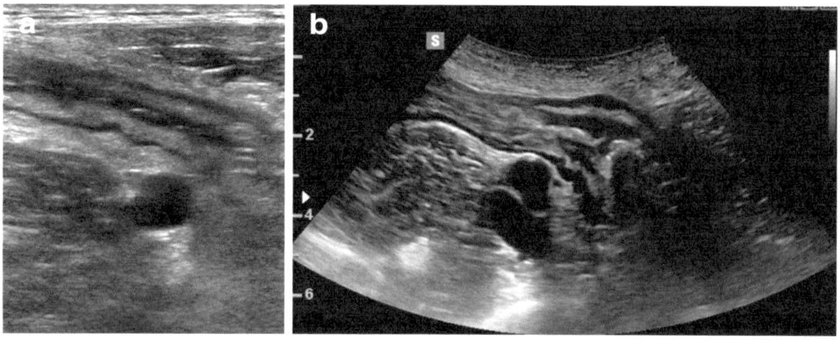

Fig. 2.5 (**a**) A demonstrates echostratification, in a thickened terminal ileum draping over the psoas muscle. The iliac artery is evident medial to the psoas muscle. There are three commonly visible layers on intestinal ultrasound, demonstrated here from the exterior of bowel wall to the interior: the hypoechoic muscularis propria, the most prominent muscle layer; the hyperechoic submucosal layer (often the most prominent layer, expanded in chronic disease states); the inner hypoechoic demonstrates the muscularis mucosae, the dark line evident just below the hyperechoic mucosa which is often bight with luminal air. Returning to the outer layer again, the serosa, can be seen as a very thin hyperechoic reflection on the margin of the muscularis propria. (**b**) Axial depiction of terminal ileum, demonstrating normal wall layers or echostratifcation, again from lumen to serosa including the muscularis mucosae, submucosa and muscularis propria, characterizing three typical wall layers consistently seen on ultrasound

wall stratification can be indicative of more significant active inflammation, oedema and even wall destruction (e.g. neoplastic process), while in chronic, inactive disease, the stratification, particularly the submucosa, can be enhanced.

2.4.2 Bowel Wall Thickness

Normal small and large bowel wall thickness, not including the duodenum or rectum, is ≤2 mm; however, the threshold for pathology is higher, ≤3–4 mm and ≥4 mm, respectively [38]. High interobserver agreement exists, particularly when standardized parameters are defined [43]. For example, consistency with transducer compression is recommended as bowel wall thickness can reduce with greater compression in healthy bowel, while it can also limit the ability to distinguish wall stratification. However, thickened and obstructed abnormal intestine with CD will not be compressible and visually remain unchanged. It is recommended that bowel wall thickness is best measured perpendicular to the wall from the interface between the serosa and muscularis propria to the interface between the mucosa and lumen [38] (Fig. 2.6).

2.4.3 Bowel Stricture and Dilation

Stricture is one of the most common complications of CD [44]. The sonographic definition of stricture varies [45]. Generally, consideration of both the wall and luminal function is important: stricturing of the wall is characterized by increased thickening (>4 mm), stiffness with compression, lack of affected wall motility combined with luminal narrowing and wall apposition (Fig. 2.7) [45]. Echostratification

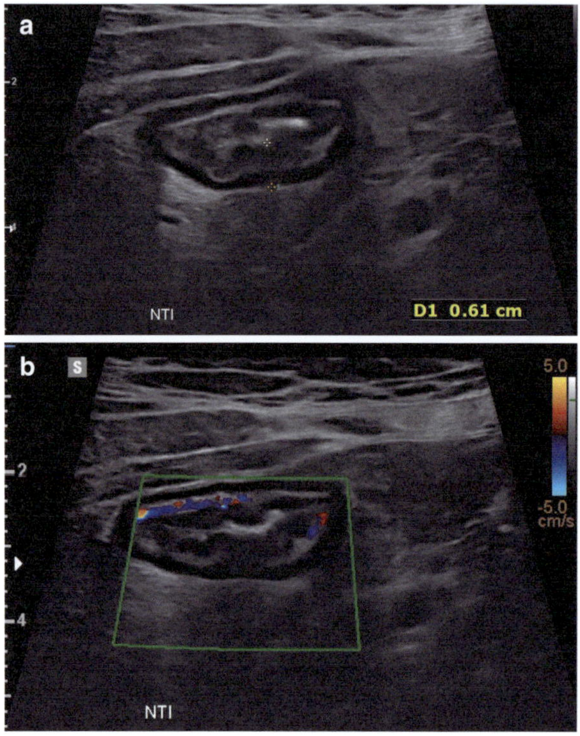

Fig. 2.6 A 36-year-old woman with moderate terminal ileal Crohn's disease, assessment of activity in transverse orientation, right lower quadrant, with measurement of the bowel wall (**a**) demonstrating increase thickening at 6.1 mm, maintenance of normal echostratification, with moderate (Lindberg 3) blood flow as demonstrated by colour Doppler signal (**b**)

may or may not be disrupted. The consequent proximal motility may be variable, with immediate proximal dilatation or absence, with associated abnormal or dysfunctional peristalsis (nonpropulsive) and/or luminal content stasis and swirling of bowel contents attempting to traverse the stricture, accompanied by increased peristalsis. Proximal loops are also important to evaluate, as upstream dilatation and abnormal peristalsis may also exist. The concurrent pre-stenotic dilation is important to characterize, as well as proximal dilatation defined as >25–30 mm in diameter, and can be underestimated during fasting [46].

2.4.4 Surrounding Mesenteric Structures

The detection of mesenteric fibrofatty proliferation is indicative of active inflammation and is characterized by a hyperechoic halo-like or "creeping fat" appearance surrounding the involved bowel segment. This creates an echogenic "window" for the affected loop of the bowel. Inflammatory fat can also separate adjacent bowel loops. Pathologic features include mesenteric fat that extends over at least half of the circumference of the bowel loops or thickening to at least 5 mm or consistently greater than normal bowel wall thickness [7] (Fig. 2.4). While the presence

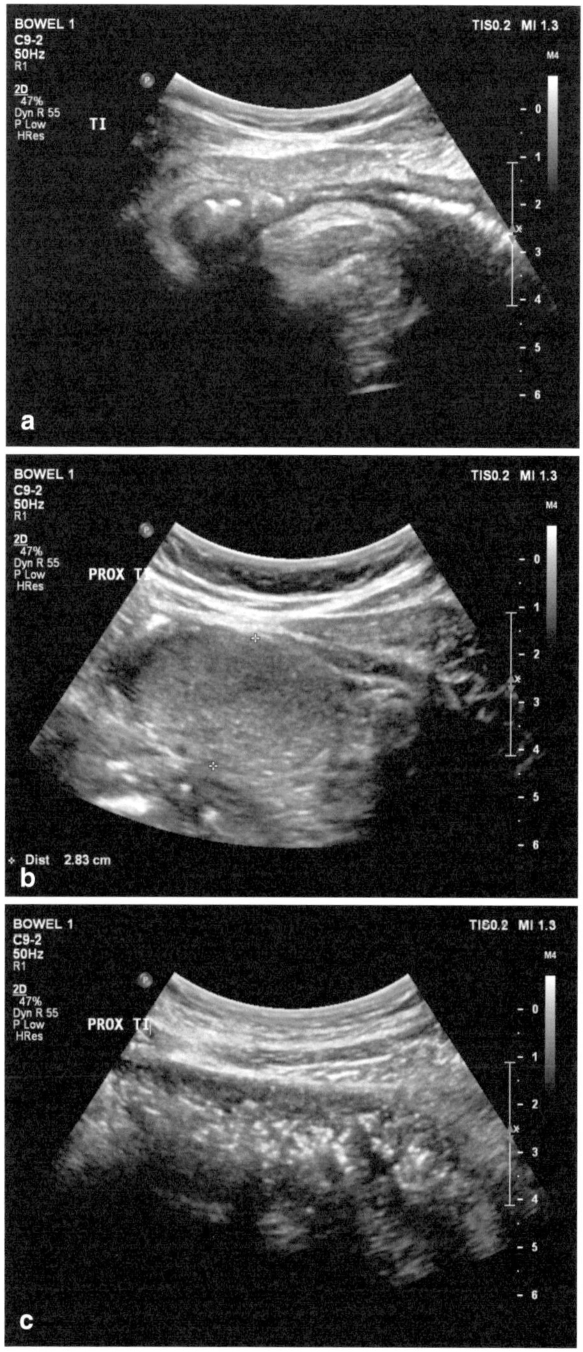

Fig. 2.7 A 56-year-old man presented with vomiting and severe abdominal pain, known long-standing ileal Crohn's disease, not currently treated as declined, in part because he had had infrequent, minimal symptoms. Intestinal ultrasound confirmed clinical suspicion of obstruction, with stricture (**a**) with proximal small bowel dilatation, dilated small bowel loops in the left upper quadrant (**b**) and the proximal terminal ileum exhibiting a "stool-like pattern" or small bowel faecalization (**c**)

of mesenteric lymphadenopathy can be associated with active disease, it is not a specific finding and may be a normal finding under 1 cm in the longitudinal axis. However, abundant, large lymph nodes can signify disease activity and should be carefully interrogated, with measurement in both long and short axis. Free fluid can be yet another ultrasonographic marker of more severe disease activity, a consequence of bowel wall oedema due to vascular and lymphatic obstruction.

2.4.5 Extra-Luminal Complications

Penetrating complications with CD are common as it is a transmural disease. Microperforations may be seen as spiculations along the serosal surface, which may subsequently develop into inflammatory masses/phlegmons or fistulae. Sonographically, a fistula is defined as a hypoechoic tract, with or without hyperechoic content, communicating between two intestinal loops or between an intestinal loop and another structure (Fig. 2.8). Gas bubbles may be seen within these tracts.

An overt perforation often leads to an abscess or a phlegmon. Abscesses are collections of pus encased in a circular wall, while phlegmons are poorly organized inflammatory masses with no obvious wall or fluid (Fig. 2.9). Phlegmons often have hyperaemia on Doppler imaging, while abscesses do not.

2.4.6 Perianal Crohn's Disease

Transperineal US of the anal canal may be valuable to assess perianal inflammation. To scan the anal canal in women, the probe is placed between the perineum and the introitus, and conversely in men, the probe is placed between the scrotum and anal canal. Fistulas, abscesses or perianal pain may be assessed with these techniques. In women, the use of endovaginal US may also be of benefit to examine perianal CD but also the rectosigmoid colon and segments of the terminal ileum found deep in the true pelvis. However, transperineal scans are limited due to patient discomfort often at the site of an open cutaneous fistula. Pelvic MRI remained the preferred test for imaging perianal CD (Chap. 9).

2.5 Contrast-Enhanced Ultrasound

Contrast-enhanced US (CEUS) involves the administration of intravenous contrast agents to dynamically evaluate the vascularity and perfusion of an organ such as the bowel [47]. Contrast-enhanced US to characterize the bowel is not routinely used, rather it remains adjunctive in some expert centres in Europe; moreover, it is currently not approved for use in the bowel in North America, and use is therefore limited. Off-label use for examination of the bowel has been approved at our centre in Canada. Contrast agents, such as Definity® and Sonovue®, consisting of lipid-coated microspheres containing microbubbles of perfluorocarbon or sulphur

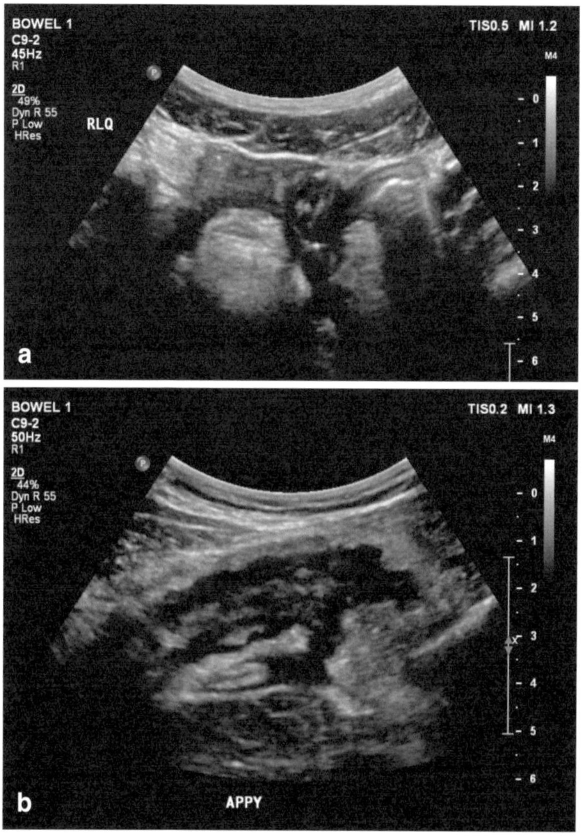

Fig. 2.8 Image from a 32-year-old male, with complex small bowel Crohn's disease, investigated given urinary tract symptoms. Transverse image with curvilinear 9–2 MHz probe, identifying penetrating terminal ileal complication, a fistula involving the sigmoid colon with air within the hypoechoic track. This is a complex image, with limited interpretative capacity in a single still image. This highlights the importance of both contribution from movie clips to better delineate anatomy, as well as the improved anatomic resolution provided by either CT or MR. (**b**) Illustrates a fistula to the appendix in a 27-year-old male with new diagnosis of ileal Crohn's disease. Note is made of loss of normal wall pattern in the distal terminal ileum, highlighting loss of echostratification

hexafluoride, respectively. Given the mean diameter of 1.1–3.3 μm, such microspheres can pass through the pulmonary vasculature to the systemic circulation, where it remains, unlike the interstitial extravasation of CT or MR contrast. The bubbles oscillate in response to US exposure; thus bubbles emit a distinct echo from surrounding tissue or vessel, which is then quantifiable, enabling perfusion level blood flow to be assessed via peak enhancement. Assessment can occur by several different methods, in either qualitative or quantitative forms. Additional parameters of assessment include the pattern of enhancement, the peak intensity of enhancement and the change in intensity over time [47].

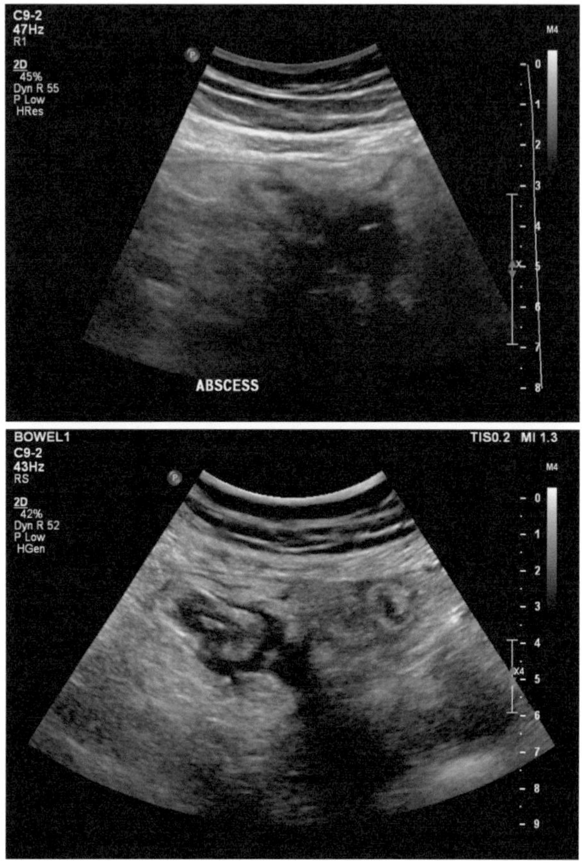

Fig. 2.9 Interloop abscess is highly suspected, with hyperechoic reflections consistent with air, surrounded by a large anechoic region, with feeding hypoechoic strands suspicious for fistulae. This patient was scanned in clinic, without access to further immediate cross-sectional imaging, so antibiotics were initiated. Further evaluation with contrast enhancement would be helpful to assess the size and potential for drainable fluid. Referral to surgery was undertaken given the failure of medical management

Roles of CEUS include characterization of bowel wall thickening with differentiation between fibrotic and inflammatory processes, as well as providing a tool to grade disease activity [48, 49]. Furthermore, CEUS can assist in assessment when there is suspicion for an abscess, by providing the ability to differentiate between vascular and avascular tissue and hence enabling differentiation of a phlegmon from an abscess [20]. A fourth indication is that of confirming and following the route of a fistula [8]. Intravenous contrast agents have an excellent safety profile, given excretion occurs through pulmonary and hepatic mechanisms; thus, use is possible in patients with renal impairment. Current evidence to support wider use of CEUS to characterize inflammation and fibrosis of the bowel is growing, with increasing evidence to support a promising quantifiable adjunct to grey scale [50].

2.5.1 Oral Contrast

Despite multiple oral contrast agents being described, there has been no clear evidence of one being superior to another, while the recommended volume and time of ingestion also remain undefined [3]. Colonic visualization can be enhanced with instillation of water, referred to as hydrocolonic ultrasound, or with oral administration of a hyperosmotic solution. The small bowel lumen however does not uniformly distend with the use of water and hyper-/hypo osmotic solutions, as water and hypo-osmolar solutions containing digestible or absorbable solutes are absorbed rapidly in the proximal small bowel, while hyperosmolar solutions with indigestible solutes delay gastric emptying and stimulate peristaltic activity [4]. Use of an iso-osmolar solution, in the form of a small quantity (ranging from 125 to 800 mL; usually 375 mL, dissolved in 250 mL of water) of polyethylene glycol (PEG), can facilitate what is regarded as small intestine contrast US (SICUS) [51]. The relatively constant gastric empting rate and subsequent retention of water in the lumen enables gradual distension throughout the small bowel [4]. Generally within 30 min, the PEG solution will have reached the terminal ileum. Extant evidence suggests improved detection of proximal small bowel lesions and complications [51–53].

2.6 Elastography

Elastography is a novel technique in IUS to assess the biomechanical elastic properties of bowel, particularly in CD where inflammation and fibrosis coexist. Quantifying the amount of fibrosis in an area of intestinal narrowing would allow management to be optimized in the form of surgical or immunosuppressant therapy. Two forms of elastography, shear wave and strain elastography, have been described in the literature. Measurements of bowel stiffness with both modalities are higher when transmural intestinal fibrosis and muscular hypertrophy are present as seen on histology of resected bowel specimens [54]. Overall, elastography is a novel and promising technique that deserves more study (see Chap. 4).

2.7 Standardized Reporting

Standardized, consistent reporting is recognized as important in imaging, to enhance consistent communication, increase quality and facilitate measurement in research [55, 56]. This is similar in other disciplines such as endoscopic, pathologic and operative reporting. Standardized reporting facilitates inclusion of crucial elements and consistency in their description and enables use of data by the referring/ordering clinician. Given concerns regarding intra and inter-rater variability, operator dependency, which is true of all modalities including endoscopy, consistent documentation is even more important in IUS. Our approach to reporting includes the following components: firstly, the quality of the study, important given potential variability in the quality of the images obtained. Poor quality studies need further cross-sectional imaging and should limit reliability/applicability of the report. Reference to prior imaging and endoscopic studies is important, with documentation of prior surgery and correlative findings. Reporting regarding activity should occur per segment reflecting activity versus normalcy, including systematic findings for the rectum; sigmoid; descending, transverse and ascending colon; caecum; terminal ileum; and small bowel including jejunum. Activity parameters include bowel wall thickness; length and distribution of bowel wall thickening; stratification preservation; mesenteric changes, in particular surrounding fibrofatty proliferation and lymphadenopathy; and hyperaemia, as measured by colour Doppler and presence of free fluid. Estimates of length with presence of skip lesions (anatomic location and number) should also be included. Clear description of location in the abdomen is important, for future replication. Then, complications including fistula(e), phlegmon, abscess, and stenosis (for each complication—outline location, size/length, anatomical involvement with neighbouring structures) need to be consistently documented. Use of oral or intravenous contrast should be outlined, with clear documentation of quality of enhancement/small bowel distention and consequent findings contrast findings as previously reported [47]. Finally, commentary on motility is important although to date, not well standardized. The presence of dilated bowel, abnormal peristalsis and content moving to and fro that is nonpropulsive are important to document. Synoptic reporting contributes significantly to ease of understanding and quick reference.

2.8 Limitations of Intestinal US

Although IUS is well tolerated by patients, with potential for easy repeatability, there are a number of important limitations to consider. Firstly, unlike other cross-sectional imaging modalities, IUS and US in general have limited anatomic resolution: without clear description of location and anatomic location in the abdomen, accurate depiction and replication of the anatomy can be challenging. This is the main argument for potential limitation in the inter- and intra-rater variability and thus reproducibility of images. This is a key limitation that may have precluded inclusion of IUS as an outcome measure in therapeutic clinical trials. However, with increasing use of both standardized assessment, documentation and synoptic reporting, as well as wider use of validated scoring systems, these limitations may be mitigated. Studies demonstrate bowel wall thickness measurements can be replicated amongst gastroenterologists at different centres with good kappa agreement scores [57]. Patients with larger body habitus and abdominal wall adiposity may hamper evaluation of the bowel; however, clinical experience is variable, and some with increased body mass index may be effectively imaged. Deep and retroperitoneal structures can be challenging, such as small bowel loops deep in pelvis and duodenum, to consistently visualize and thus characterize. Moreover, given limitations in anatomic resolution, alterations from multiple prior bowel surgeries require careful and expert interrogation of the location often with the help of prior additional imaging with CT or MR. In this circumstance, once the anatomy is mapped, IUS provides an excellent follow-up modality. Ultrasound of the bowel is often performed in centres with dedication to imaging of inflammatory bowel disease, and these challenges may be largely overcome with collaboration with experienced sonographers and radiologists.

2.9 Summary

Use of IUS has the capacity to improve the access to safe, easily repeated, objective monitoring of patients with IBD. It is comparable to alternate cross-sectional imaging and endoscopy in accuracy, with high sensitivity and specificity for detecting disease activity. Intestinal US can also be performed at the bedside by well trained, experienced gastroenterologists, providing objective information to guide clinical decision-making. This ideally occurs in close collaboration with radiology, as the cross-pollination of expertise is ideal for quality patient care. In addition to the real-time acquisition of luminal and functional characterization, this patient-centred approach enables an opportunity to engage and educate patients about their disease. Intestinal US is not without limitations; however, the development of validated scoring tools that assist in quantifying disease activity, along with a formulaic methodology for performing IUS and systematic reporting of findings, will mitigate these commonly perceived limitations.

References

1. Holt S, Samuel E. Grey scale ultrasound in Crohn's disease. Gut. 1979;20(7):590–5.
2. Daperno M, Castiglione F, de Ridder L, Dotan I, Färkkilä M, Florholmen J, et al. Results of the 2nd part scientific workshop of the ECCO. II: measures and markers of prediction to achieve, detect, and monitor intestinal healing in inflammatory bowel disease. J Crohns Colitis. 2011;5(5):484–98.
3. Peyrin-Biroulet L, Reinisch W, Colombel J-F, Mantzaris GJ, Kornbluth A, Diamond R, et al. Clinical disease activity, C-reactive protein normalisation and mucosal healing in Crohn's disease in the SONIC trial. Gut. 2014;63(1):88–95.
4. Bouguen G, Levesque BG, Feagan BG, Kavanaugh A, Peyrin-Biroulet L, Colombel J-F, et al. Treat to target: a proposed new paradigm for the management of Crohn's disease. Clin Gastroenterol Hepatol. 2015;13(6):1042–50.e2.
5. Greenup A, Bressler B, Rosenfeld G. Medical imaging in small bowel Crohn's disease—computed tomography enterography, magnetic resonance enterography, and ultrasound:"which one is the best for what?". Inflamm Bowel Dis. 2016;22(5):1246–61.
6. Panés J, Bouzas R, Chaparro M, García-Sánchez V, Gisbert JP, Martínez de Guereñu B, et al. Systematic review: the use of ultrasonography, computed tomography and magnetic resonance imaging for the diagnosis, assessment of activity and abdominal complications of Crohn's disease. Aliment Pharmacol Ther. 2011;34(2):125–45.
7. Calabrese E, Maaser C, Zorzi F, Kannengiesser K, Hanauer SB, Bruining DH, et al. Bowel ultrasonography in the management of Crohn's disease. A review with recommendations of an international panel of experts. Inflamm Bowel Dis. 2016;22(5):1168–83.
8. Fraquelli M, Casazza G, Paggi S, Colucci A, Massironi S, Duca P, et al. Role of US in detection of Crohn disease: meta-analysis. Radiology. 2005;236:95–101.
9. Horsthuis K, Bipat S, Bennink R, Stoker J. Inflammatory bowel disease diagnosed with US, MR, scintigraphy, and CT: meta-analysis of prospective studies. Radiology. 2008;247(1):64–79.
10. Zhu C, Ma X, Xue L, Xu J, Li Q, Wang Y, et al. Small intestine contrast ultrasonography for the detection and assessment of Crohn disease: a meta-analysis. Medicine (Baltimore). 2016;95(31):e4235.
11. Peyrin-Biroulet L, Sandborn W, Sands BE, Reinisch W, Bemelman W, Bryant RV, et al. Selecting therapeutic targets in inflammatory bowel disease (STRIDE): determining therapeutic goals for treat-to-target. Am J Gastroenterol. 2015;110(9):1324–38.

12. Moreno N, Ripollés T, Paredes JM, Ortiz I, Martínez MJ, López A, et al. Usefulness of abdominal ultrasonography in the analysis of endoscopic activity in patients with Crohn's disease: changes following treatment with immunomodulators and/or anti-TNF antibodies. J Crohns Colitis. 2014;8(9):1079–87.
13. Fernandes SR, Rodrigues RV, Bernardo S, Cortez-Pinto J, Rosa I, Da Silva JP, et al. Transmural healing is associated with improved long-term outcomes of patients with Crohn's disease. Inflamm Bowel Dis. 2017;23(8):1403–9.
14. Castiglione F, Testa A, Rea M, De Palma GD, Diaferia M, Musto D, et al. Transmural healing evaluated by bowel sonography in patients with Crohn's disease on maintenance treatment with biologics. Inflamm Bowel Dis. 2013;19(9):1928–34.
15. Castiglione F, Mainenti P, Testa A, Imperatore N, De Palma GD, Maurea S, et al. Cross-sectional evaluation of transmural healing in patients with Crohn's disease on maintenance treatment with anti-TNF alpha agents. Dig Liver Dis. 2017;49(5):484–9.
16. Dillman JR, Dehkordy SF, Smith EA, DiPietro MA, Sanchez R, DeMatos-Maillard V, et al. Defining the ultrasound longitudinal natural history of newly diagnosed pediatric small bowel Crohn disease treated with infliximab and infliximab–azathioprine combination therapy. Pediatr Radiol. Pediatr Radiol. 2017;47(8):924–34.
17. Ripollés T, Paredes JM, Martínez-Pérez MJ, Rimola J, Jauregui-Amezaga A, Bouzas R, et al. Ultrasonographic changes at 12 weeks of anti-TNF drugs predict 1-year sonographic response and clinical outcome in Crohn's disease: a multicenter study. Inflamm Bowel Dis. 2016;22(10):2465–73.
18. Deepak P, Fletcher JG, Fidler JL, Barlow JM, Sheedy SP, Kolbe AB, et al. Radiological response is associated with better long-term outcomes and is a potential treatment target in patients with small bowel Crohn's disease. Am J Gastroenterol. 2016;111(7):997–1006.
19. Rispo A, Imperatore N, Testa A, Mainenti P, De Palma GD, Luglio G, et al. Bowel damage in Crohn's disease: direct comparison of ultrasonography-based and magnetic resonance-based lemann index. Inflamm Bowel Dis. 2017;23(1):143–51.
20. Ripollés T, Martínez-Pérez MJ, Paredes JM, Vizuete J, García-Martínez E, Jiménez-Restrepo DH. Contrast-enhanced ultrasound in the differentiation between phlegmon and abscess in crohn's disease and other abdominal conditions. Eur J Radiol. 2013;82(10):e525–31.
21. Zorzi F, Stasi E, Bevivino G, Scarozza P, Biancone L, Zuzzi S, et al. A sonographic lesion index for Crohn's disease helps monitor changes in transmural bowel damage during therapy. Clin Gastroenterol Hepatol. 2014;12(12):2071–7.
22. Onali S, Calabrese E, Petruzziello C, Lolli E, Ascolani M, Ruffa A, et al. Post-operative recurrence of Crohn's disease: a prospective study at 5 years. Dig Liver Dis. 2016; 48(5):489–94.
23. Calabrese E, Petruzziello C, Onali S, Condino G, Zorzi F, Pallone F, et al. Severity of postoperative recurrence in Crohn's disease: correlation between endoscopic and sonographic findings. Inflamm Bowel Dis. 2009;15(11):1635–42.
24. Paredes JM, Ripollés T, Cortés X, Moreno N, Martínez MJ, Bustamante-Balén M, et al. Contrast-enhanced ultrasonography: usefulness in the assessment of postoperative recurrence of Crohn's disease. J Crohns Colitis. 2013;7(3):192–201.
25. Wright EK, Novak KL, Lu C, Panaccione R, Ghosh S, Wilson SR. Transperineal ultrasonography in perianal Crohn disease: a valuable imaging modality. Can J Gastroenterol Hepatol. 2015;29(8):445–7.
26. Maconi G, Ardizzone S, Greco S, Radice E, Bezzio C, Bianchi Porro G. Transperineal ultrasound in the detection of perianal and rectovaginal fistulae in Crohn's disease. Am J Gastroenterol. 2007;102(10):2214–9.
27. Molodecky NA, Soon IS, Rabi DM, Ghali WA, Ferris M, Chernoff G, et al. Increasing incidence and prevalence of the inflammatory bowel diseases with time, based on systematic review. Gastroenterology. 2012;142(1):46–54.e42.
28. Huang JS, Tobin A, Harvey L, Nelson TR. Diagnostic medical radiation in pediatric patients with inflammatory bowel disease. J Pediatr Gastroenterol Nutr. 2011;53(5):502–6.

29. Levine A, Koletzko S, Turner D, Escher JC, Cucchiara S, De Ridder L, et al. ESPGHAN revised Porto criteria for the diagnosis of inflammatory bowel disease in children and adolescents. J Pediatr Gastroenterol Nutr. 2014;58(6):795–806.
30. Yoon H, Suh C, Kim J, Lee J, Jung A, Kim K, et al. Diagnostic performance of magnetic resonance enterography for detection of active inflammation in children and adolescents with inflammatory bowel disease a systematic review and diagnostic meta-analysis. JAMA Pediatr. 2017;171(12):1208–16.
31. Borthne AS, Abdelnoor M, Rugtveit J, Perminow G, Reiseter T, Kløw NE. Bowel magnetic resonance imaging of pediatric patients with oral mannitol: MRI compared to endoscopy and intestinal ultrasound. Eur Radiol. 2006;16(1):207–14.
32. Tsai TL, Marine MB, Wanner MR, Cooper ML, Steiner SJ, Ouyang F, et al. Can ultrasound be used as the primary imaging in children with suspected Crohn disease? Pediatr Radiol. 2017;47(8):917–23.
33. Pallotta N, Civitelli F, Di Nardo G, Vincoli G, Aloi M, Viola F, et al. Small intestine contrast ultrasonography in pediatric crohn's disease. J Pediatr. 2013;163(3):778–84.
34. Civitelli F, Di Nardo G, Oliva S, Nuti F, Ferrari F, Dilillo A, et al. Ultrasonography of the colon in pediatric ulcerative colitis: a prospective, blind, comparative study with colonoscopy. J Pediatr. 2014;165(1):78–84.e2.
35. Parente F, Molteni M, Marino B, Colli A, Ardizzone S, Greco S, et al. Are colonoscopy and bowel ultrasound useful for assessing response to short-term therapy and predicting disease outcome of moderate-to-severe forms of ulcerative colitis: a prospective study. Am J Gastroenterol. 2010;105(5):1150–7.
36. Kucharzik T, Kannengiesser K, Petersen F. The use of ultrasound in in fl ammatory bowel disease. Ann Gastroenterol. 2017;30(2):135–44.
37. Parente F, Molteni M, Marino B, Colli A, Ardizzone S, Greco S, Sampietro GGS. Bowel ultrasound and mucosal healing in ulcerative colitis. Dig Dis. 2009;27:285–90.
38. Nylund K, Maconi G, Hollerweger A, Ripolles T, Pallotta N, Higginson A, et al. EFSUMB recommendations and guidelines for gastrointestinal ultrasound - part 1: examination techniques and normal findings (long version). Ultraschall Med. 2017;38(3):e1–e15.
39. Ung C, Chang ST, Brooke Jeffrey R, Patel BN, Olcott EW. Sonography of the normal appendix: its varied appearance and techniques to improve its visualization. Ultrasound Q. 2013;29(4):333–41.
40. Deslandes A. Sonographic demonstration of stomach pathology: reviewing the cases. Australas J Ultrasound Med. 2013;16(4):202–9. https://doi.org/10.1002/j.2205-0140.2013.tb00249.x.
41. Taylor SA, Avni F, Cronin CG, Hoeffel C, Kim SH, Laghi A, et al. The first joint ESGAR/ESPR consensus statement on the technical performance of cross-sectional small bowel and colonic imaging. Eur Radiol. 2017;27(6):2570–82.
42. Limberg B. Diagnosis of acute ulcerative colitis and colonic Crohn's disease by colonic sonography. J Clin Ultrasound. 1989;17(1):25–31.
43. Fraquelli M, Sarno a GC, Laudi C, Buscarini E, Villa C, et al. Reproducibility of bowel ultrasonography in the evaluation of Crohn's disease. Dig Liver Dis. 2008;40(11):860–6.
44. Rieder F, Latella G, Magro F, Yuksel ES, Higgins PDR, Di Sabatino A, et al. European Crohn's and colitis organisation topical review on prediction, diagnosis and management of fibrostenosing Crohn's disease. J Crohns Colitis. 2016;10(8):873–85.
45. Coelho R, Ribeiro H, Maconi G. Bowel thickening in Crohn's disease: fibrosis or inflammation? Diagnostic ultrasound imaging tools. Inflamm Bowel Dis. 2017;23(1):23–34.
46. Silva AC, Pimenta M, Guimarães LS. Small bowel obstruction: what to look for. Radiographics. 2009;29(2):423–39.
47. Medellin A, Merrill C, Wilson SR. Role of contrast-enhanced ultrasound in evaluation of the bowel. Abdom Radiol (NY). 2018;43(4):918–33.
48. Quaia E, De Paoli L, Stocca T, Cabibbo B, Casagrande F, Cova MA. The value of small bowel wall contrast enhancement after sulfur hexafluoride-filled microbubble injection to differentiate inflammatory from fibrotic strictures in patients with Crohn's disease. Ultrasound Med Biol. 2012;38(8):1324–32.

49. Quaia E, Gennari AG, Cova MA, van Beek EJR. Differentiation of inflammatory from fibrotic ileal strictures among patients with Crohn's disease based on visual analysis: feasibility study combining conventional B-mode ultrasound, contrast-enhanced ultrasound and strain elastography. Ultrasound Med Biol. 2018;44(4):762–70.
50. Wilkens R, Hagemann-Madsen RH, Peters DA, Nielsen AH, Nørager CB, Glerup H, et al. Validity of contrast enhanced ultrasonography and dynamic contrast enhanced MR Enterography in the assessment of transmural activity and fibrosis in Crohn's disease. J Crohns Colitis. 2018;12(1):48–56.
51. Pallotta N, Vincoli G, Montesani C, Chirletti P, Pronio A, Caronna R, et al. Small intestine contrast ultrasonography (SICUS) for the detection of small bowel complications in crohn's disease: a prospective comparative study versus intraoperative findings. Inflamm Bowel Dis. 2012;18(1):74–84.
52. Onali S, Calabrese E, Petruzziello C, Zorzi F, Sica G, Fiori R, et al. Small intestine contrast ultrasonography vs computed tomography enteroclysis for assessing ileal Crohn's disease. World J Gastroenterol. 2012;18(42):6088–95.
53. Calabrese E, Zorzi F, Onali S, Petruzziello C, Condino G, Lolli E, et al. Small intestine contrast ultrasonography for detecting asymptomatic small bowel Crohn's disease lesions: a family study. Dig Liver Dis. 2011;43:S210–1.
54. Havre R, Gilja OH. Elastography and strain rate imaging of the gastrointestinal tract. Eur J Radiol. 2014;83(3):438–41.
55. Wildman-tobriner B, Allen BC, Bashir MR, Camp M, Miller C, Fiorillo LE, et al. Structured reporting of CT enterography for inflammatory bowel disease : effect on key feature reporting, accuracy across training levels, and subjective assessment of disease by referring physicians. Abdom Radiol (NY). 2017;42(9):2243–50.
56. Bruining DH, Zimmermann EM, Loftus EV, Sandborn WJ, Sauer CG, Strong SA. Consensus recommendations for evaluation, interpretation, and utilization of computed tomography and magnetic resonance enterography in patients with small bowel Crohn's disease. Gastroenterology. 2018;154(4):1172–94.
57. Kucharzik T, Wittig BM, Helwig U, Börner N, Rössler A, Rath S, et al. Use of intestinal ultrasound to monitor Crohn's disease activity. Clin Gastroenterol Hepatol. 2017;15(4):535–542.e2.

Ultrasound Elastography of the Bowel

3

Jonathan R. Dillman, Jonathan M. Rubin, Laura A. Johnson, and Peter D.R. Higgins

Abstract

Over the past decade, there has been increasing evidence that ultrasound elastography may aid in the imaging evaluation and management of pediatric and adult Crohn's disease patients. Multiple studies have shown that ultrasound-derived intestinal stiffness measurements can suggest the presence of bowel wall fibrosis in areas of stricturing disease, even in the setting of superimposed inflammation. Such knowledge can help guide the appropriate medical and surgical management of these patients. Furthermore, semiquantitative and quantitative elastographic methods may predict response to medical therapy, show evidence of progressive bowel damage over time, and potentially predict ensuing complications, such as impending bowel obstruction or penetrating complications. This chapter will review the different ultrasound elastography techniques for assessing the bowel, published evidence supporting the use of these techniques in Crohn's disease patients, potential roles in clinical practice, and likely challenges and obstacles to future clinical use.

J. R. Dillman (✉)
Department of Radiology, Cincinnati Children's Hospital Medical Center, Cincinnati, OH, USA
e-mail: jonathan.dillman@cchmc.org

J. M. Rubin
Department of Radiology, University of Michigan/Michigan Medicine, Ann Arbor, MI, USA

L. A. Johnson · P. D.R. Higgins
Department of Internal Medicine, Division of Gastroenterology and Hepatology, University of Michigan/Michigan Medicine, Ann Arbor, MI, USA

J. Rimola (ed.), *Cross-Sectional Imaging in Crohn's Disease*,
https://doi.org/10.1007/978-3-319-96586-4_3

3.1 Introduction

Ultrasound has multiple roles in the evaluation of children and adults with Crohn's disease. Common uses include the detection of affected bowel segments, assessment of intestinal inflammation, and evaluation of response to medical therapy [1–3]. Ultrasound also can be used to evaluate for intra-abdominal complications of Crohn's disease, including fistulas, phlegmons (also known as inflammatory masses), and abscesses [1, 4].

Another application of ultrasound in the setting of Crohn's disease relates to detecting and characterizing areas of bowel wall thickening and luminal narrowing that may be associated with variable intestinal obstruction, so-called stricturing disease (Fig. 3.1). It is likely that many Crohn's disease patients progress from (1) simple intestinal inflammation without luminal narrowing to (2) considerable wall thickening with luminal narrowing to (3) considerable wall thickening and luminal narrowing with more proximal (upstream) bowel dilatation (i.e., a stricture) [5]. Narrowed, obstructing bowel segments may demonstrate inflammation (active and/or chronic), fibrosis, smooth muscle hypertrophy, or some combination of these

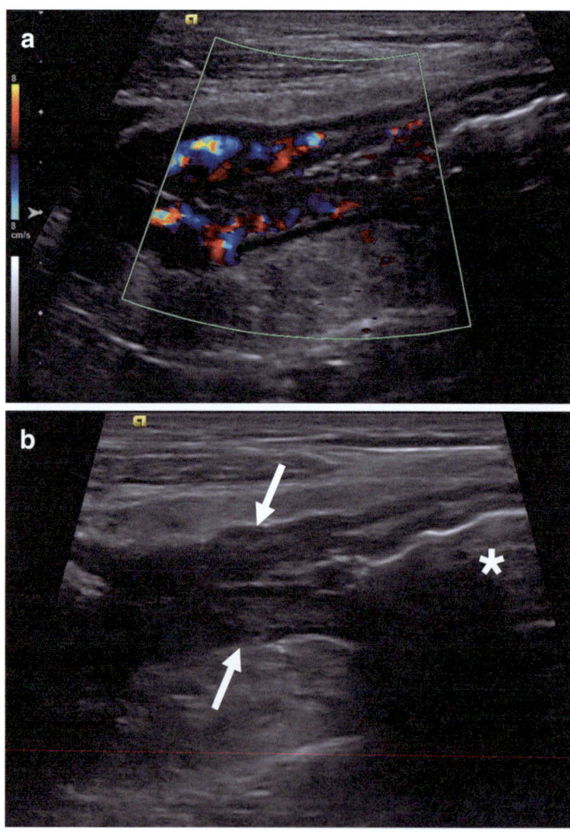

Fig. 3.1 Teenage boy with stricturing Crohn's disease. (**a**) Longitudinal color Doppler image of the terminal ileum shows bowel wall thickening and luminal narrowing. There is mildly increased blood flow in the bowel wall due to inflammation, and adjacent echogenic tissue is consistent with thickened, fatty mesentery. (**b**) Another longitudinal gray-scale image shows terminal ileal wall thickening and luminal narrowing (*arrows*) with more proximal small bowel dilatation (*asterisk*), consistent with stricturing disease

upon histopathologic evaluation [6]. Different recent studies suggest that obstructing strictures almost always are histologically mixed, containing both inflammation and fibrosis [7–9].

While conventional gray-scale and Doppler ultrasound techniques can be used to identify intestinal strictures and confirm the presence of inflammation, the existence of fibrosis within a stricture has been more challenging to detect. As an example, a stricture showing marked color or power Doppler hyperemia can be associated with no, mild, or severe mural fibrosis. Currently, patients with strictures with no or mild fibrosis may positively respond to medical (i.e., anti-inflammatory or immunosuppressive) therapy, while patients with strictures with severe fibrosis almost certainly would benefit from an endoscopic (e.g., balloon dilatation) or surgical (e.g., stricturoplasty or resection) intervention as medical management is unlikely to have an enduring result with long-term relief of intestinal obstruction [10, 11].

Over the past decade, there is increasing evidence that ultrasound elastography of the bowel may help meet this unmet need. That is, ultrasound elasticity (stiffness) imaging may suggest the presence of bowel wall fibrosis in strictures, even in the setting of substantial active inflammation. Furthermore, semiquantitative and quantitative elastography methods may estimate the severity of intestinal fibrosis and allow assessment of change over time, thus guiding medical and surgical management and predicting impending complications.

3.2 Imaging Techniques

Ultrasound elastographic methods have the potential to be a rapid, noninvasive, well-tolerated nonionizing method for detecting, measuring, and following intestinal injury and fibrosis over time. Elastography is a radiologic analog to manual palpation, where the hands are used to physically examine the body (or the intestine during surgery) and feel for areas of abnormal hardness. There are two basic ultrasound techniques for assessing tissue stiffness: (1) strain-based elastography and (2) shear wave-based elastography.

3.2.1 Ultrasound Strain Elastography

Strain-based elastographic methods typically characterize tissue using gray-scale speckle (echo) tracking to establish stiffness based on how a particular tissue responds to ultrasound transducer pressure (stress) [12, 13]. Simply put, softer tissues (e.g., inflamed bowel without substantial fibrosis) deform readily in response to stress and thus demonstrate high strain, whereas harder tissues (e.g., bowel wall with substantial fibrosis with or without inflammation) show minimal deformation and instead translate or displace with stress and thus demonstrate low strain.

Strain elastography techniques that are available on most state-of-the-art ultrasound systems are semiquantitative, providing color maps (elastograms) of relative stiffness and allowing estimates of stiffness using strain ratios, where the

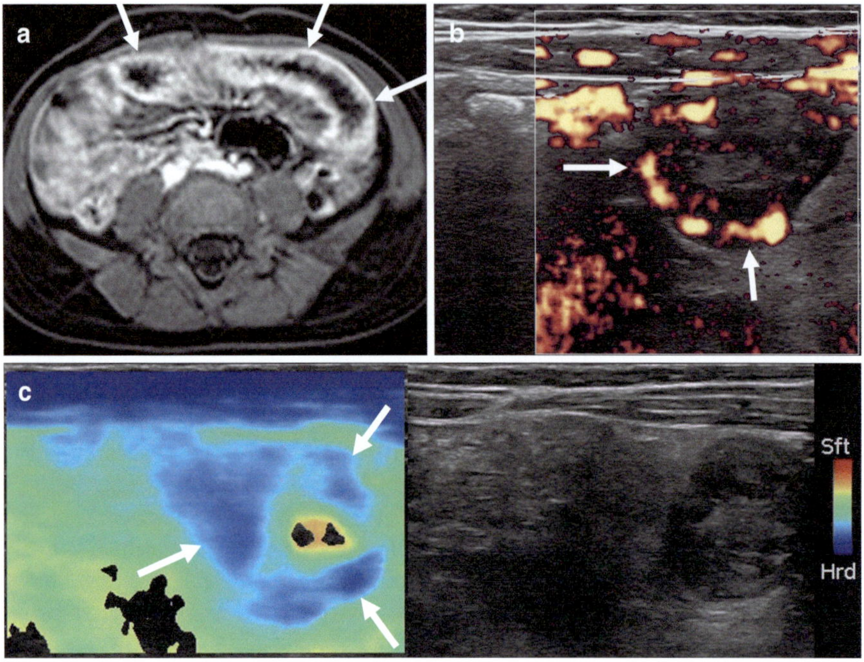

Fig. 3.2 A 6-year-old girl with newly diagnosed Crohn's disease. (**a**) Axial postcontrast T1-weighted fat-suppressed MR image shows extensive jejunal wall thickening and mural hyper-enhancement (*arrows*), consistent with active inflammation. Mesenteric vascular structures are engorged. (**b**) Power Doppler image of the left anterior abdomen shows a thick-walled small bowel loop (*arrows*) with associated mural and mesenteric hyperemia. Adjacent mesenteric fat appears thickened. (**c**) Strain elastography stiffness map (elastogram) with side-by-side gray-scale image shows that the bowel wall (*arrows*) is substantially harder than adjacent mesentery (blue is hard and red is soft)

tissue of interest is normalized to an adjacent (often assumed to be normal) tissue (Fig. 3.2). Strain ratios >1 are indicative of tissue stiffening. The operator may exert manual compression or hold the transducer steady and rely on physiologic motion (i.e., breathing) in order to apply stress (so-called quasi-static strain elastography) [13].

3.2.2 Ultrasound Shear Wave Elastography

More recently, ultrasound shear wave-based elastographic methods have become available. These techniques are based on the generation of in vivo shear waves in the thickened bowel wall using focused ultrasound (acoustic radiation force impulse [i.e., ARFI]) and measurement of their speed as they propagate transversely [13–15]. Measured shear wave speed increases with increasing material (tissue) stiffness. Shear wave speed can be related to Young's modulus (kPa) (e.g., after making basic assumptions regarding tissue density, boundary conditions, and isotropy), a mechanical property of linear elastic solid materials that defines the relationship between stress (or force/area) and strain (or deformation) [14, 15].

Both point and two-dimensional (2D) shear wave elastography techniques are available, where the point method excites a single focal anatomic location and the 2D method uses multiple "push pulses" in rapid sequence to create a shear wave-based elastogram (Fig. 3.3) [13]. Shear wave elastography cannot be used to interrogate normal bowel wall, as the bowel wall is too thin to reliably track and measure the speed of shear waves which have a considerably longer wavelength than the bowel wall thickness.

3.3 Supporting Studies

3.3.1 Ultrasound Strain Elastography

Using the trinitrobenzenesulfonic acid (TNBS) rodent model that recapitulates the bowel wall inflammation and fibrosis of human Crohn's disease, Kim et al. [16] initially demonstrated that ultrasound strain elastography allowed characterization of local bowel wall elastic properties. Specifically, strain measurements differentiated diseased fibrotic intestine from normal intestine based on histology as well as direct mechanical measurement of tissue stiffness. This same research group went on to describe a novel nonlinear strain elastography method also in rodents that measured change in developed bowel wall strain as a function of increasing applied stress (based on overall abdominal strain) [17]. Based on this relationship (curve), a continuous nonlinear parameter was generated that in theory has a considerably larger dynamic range than conventional quasi-static strain elastography. This nonlinear parameter was able to reliably differentiate normal intestine from acutely inflamed intestine and acutely inflamed intestine from fibrotic intestine.

In a small pilot study, Havre et al. [18] used ultrasound strain elastography to assess 16 freshly resected stenotic Crohn's disease lesions. These authors showed that the abnormal bowel wall was harder than surrounding tissues. Baumgart et al. [19] also used strain elastography to assess Crohn's disease strictures as well as normal intestine both in vivo and ex vivo. In this study of ten patients, there was a good correlation between preoperative, intraoperative, and postoperative (i.e., in vivo and ex vivo) strain values obtained from both unaffected and affected bowel segments and that there were significant differences in strain measurements between unaffected and strictured intestine. Furthermore, strain measurements correlated with bowel wall collagen content, a marker of tissue fibrosis.

Fraquelli et al. [20] performed ultrasound strain elastography in 23 Crohn's disease patients undergoing resection of the terminal ileum as well as in 20 patients with uncomplicated inflammatory terminal ileitis. Strain ratios were shown to significantly correlate with both semiquantitative and quantitative histological assessments of the resected intestine. These measurements had

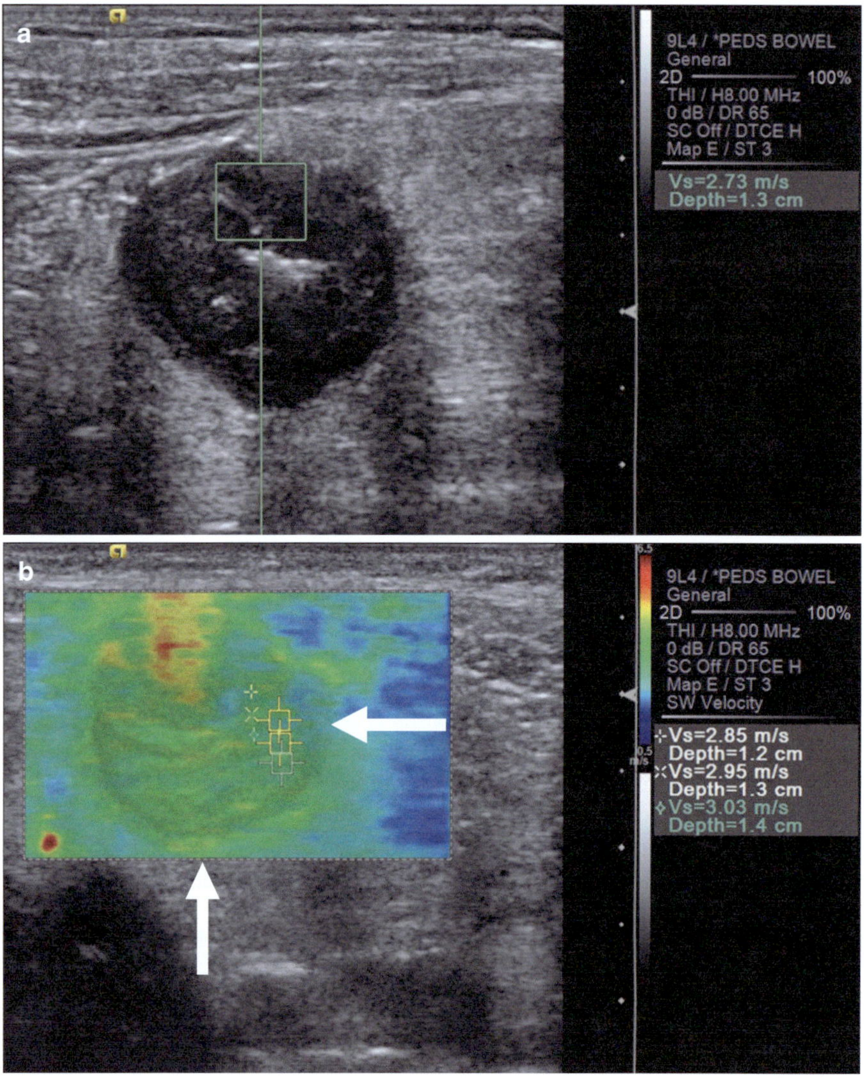

Fig. 3.3 A 13-year-old boy with Crohn's disease. (**a**) There are marked terminal ileal wall thickening, luminal narrowing, and adjacent mesenteric fatty thickening. Point ultrasound shear wave elastography assessment shows abnormal bowel wall stiffening at the 12 o'clock location, with a measured shear wave speed of 2.73 m/s. (**b**) 2D shear wave elastography elastogram also demonstrates abnormal stiffening of the bowel wall (*arrows*) when compared to adjacent mesentery. Three shear wave speed measurements at the 3 o'clock location range from 2.85 to 3.03 m/s

excellent diagnostic performance for detecting severe bowel wall fibrosis (area-under-the-receiver operator characteristic curve = 0.92) and demonstrated excellent inter-rater agreement. Strain ratios also were significantly different when comparing operated Crohn's disease patients to individuals with uncomplicated inflammatory disease.

In a systematic review of bowel ultrasound strain elastography by Pescatori et al. [21], a total of 7 articles were identified that included 129 patients and 154 small and large bowel lesions. In all of these studies, the authors found that elastography results correlated with intestinal fibrosis and that bowel wall strain significantly decreases in fibrotic strictures. These authors also concluded that while the various articles were rather heterogeneous and challenging to compare, ultrasound strain elastography is a "promising tool" for identifying bowel wall fibrosis in Crohn's disease patients.

Finally, ultrasound strain elastography has been shown to predict therapeutic outcomes in Crohn's disease patients treated with biologic therapy. In a study by Orlando et al. [22], 30 consecutive patients with ileal or ileocolonic Crohn's disease starting antitumor necrosis factor therapy underwent strain elastography of the bowel at baseline and 14 and 52 weeks. Using strain ratios between the bowel wall and adjacent mesentery, the need for surgery was significantly higher in patients with a strain ratio ≥ 2 at baseline ($p = 0.003$). Baseline strain ratios also were significantly lower in patients that experienced transmural healing.

3.3.2 Ultrasound Shear Wave Elastography

There is a substantially smaller number of animal and human studies using ultrasound shear wave elastography to evaluate intestinal fibrosis. Using 2D shear wave elastography and the TNBS rodent model, Dillman et al. [23] documented higher bowel wall shear wave speeds in inflamed versus fibrotic bowel segments (Fig. 3.4). This difference in shear wave speeds increased with increasing transducer preload (stress). The shear wave speed to stress (based on developed abdominal strain from ultrasound transducer pressure) ratio was accurate for differentiating histologically fibrotic from inflamed bowel segments (area-under-the-receiver operating characteristic curve = 0.97).

In a small pilot study, the same authors [24] used both point and 2D shear wave elastographic methods to assess the elastic properties of 17 freshly resected bowel segments (15 small and 2 large intestine) from Crohn's disease patients, confirming that shear wave speed measurements increase with increasing mural fibrosis (Figs. 3.5 and 3.6). Ex vivo imaging was performed on the specimens at the 9 o'clock, 12 o'clock, and 3 o'clock locations in the areas of most severe stricturing. Bowel segments with transmural fibrosis had significantly higher mean shear wave speed measurements than bowel segments with lesser fibrosis (1.59 vs. 1.18 m/s using point and 1.87 vs. 1.50 m/s using 2D shear wave elastography, respectively).

In a prospective study of 105 consecutive patients with ileal Crohn's disease, Lu et al. [6] performed ultrasound shear wave elastography in areas of wall thickening greater than 4 mm. Fifteen of these patients underwent ileal resection within an average of 71 days with regard to ultrasound imaging. Mean bowel wall shear wave speed was significantly higher in patients with versus without surgery (2.8 vs. 2.2 m/s). Interestingly, these authors concluded that the bowel wall stiffening seen in Crohn's disease may be primarily due to smooth muscle hypertrophy as opposed

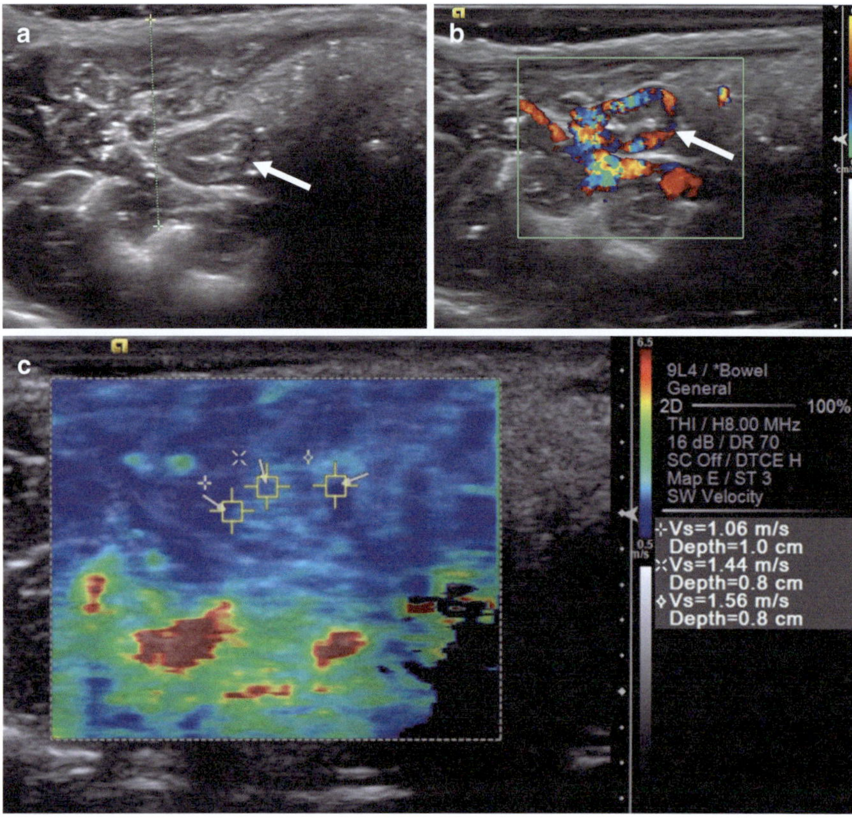

Fig. 3.4 Ultrasound shear wave elastography of acutely inflamed bowel in the TNBS rodent model of Crohn's disease. (**a**) Transverse gray-scale ultrasound image shows thick-walled sigmoid colon (*arrow*). (**b**) Color Doppler image shows marked bowel wall hyperemia (*arrow*) due to active inflammation. (**c**) 2D shear wave elastography elastogram shows that the bowel wall stiffness is similar to adjacent mesentery and not abnormally stiffened (shear wave speed range, 1.06–1.56 m/s)

to fibrosis based on a moderate positive correlation between shear wave speed and muscular hypertrophy ($r = 0.59$) and no statistically significant relationship between shear wave speed and histopathologic fibrosis.

3.4 Potential Roles of Ultrasound Elastography of the Bowel in Clinical Practice

While the roles of ultrasound elastography of the bowel in Crohn's disease have yet to be clearly defined, there are several promising applications. First and perhaps most useful, assessment of bowel wall stiffness can likely be used to determine the presence versus absence of substantial fibrosis in stricturing lesions, even when inflammation is coexistent (Fig. 3.7). Ultrasound can potentially provide an

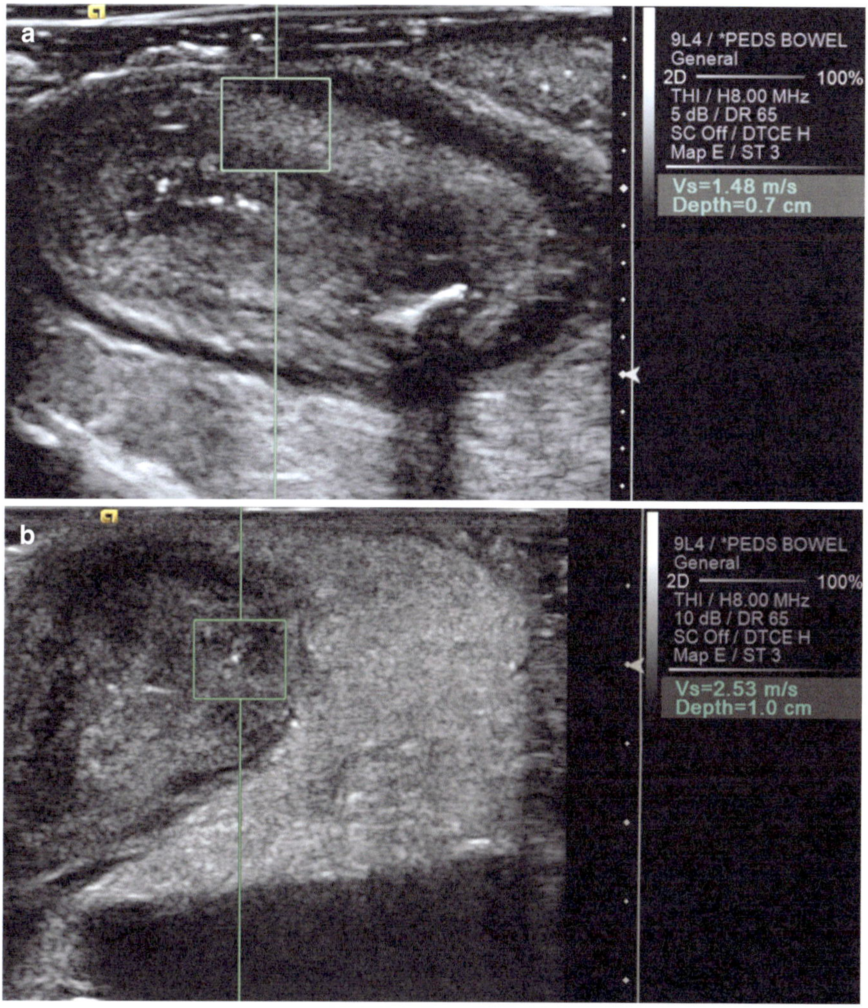

Fig. 3.5 Point shear wave elastography images of freshly resected terminal ileal small bowel specimens from two different teenage Crohn's disease patients. Both patients show substantial bowel wall thickening and mesenteric fatty proliferation (**a**) Shear wave speed measurement was 1.48 m/s at the 12 o'clock position in the first patient, which suggests minimal bowel wall stiffening and likely negligible fibrosis. (**b**) Shear wave speed measurement was 2.53 m/s at the 3 o'clock position in the second patient, which suggests substantial bowel wall stiffening and likely transmural fibrosis

"acoustic biopsy" of the bowel wall and guide medical versus surgical management or endoscopic dilatation, as stenotic lesions with considerable fibrosis and muscular hypertrophy are unlikely to have an enduring response to medical treatment. Such information also may allow more frequent non-emergent surgical interventions, thereby decreasing surgical complications that can occur when surgery is emergent and lowering healthcare costs.

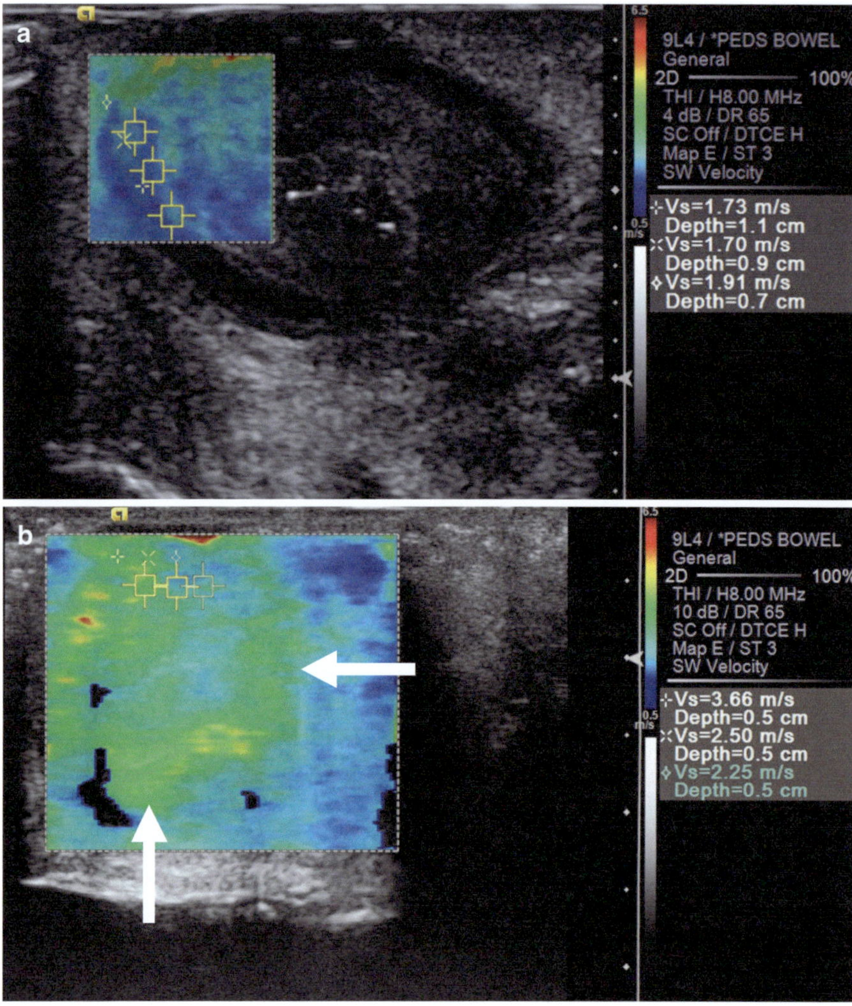

Fig. 3.6 2D shear wave elastography images of freshly resected terminal ileal small bowel specimens from two different teenage Crohn's disease patients. Both patients show substantial bowel wall thickening and mesenteric fatty proliferation (**a**) Shear wave speed measurements ranged from 1.70 to 1.91 m/s at the 9 o'clock position in the first patient. (**b**) Shear wave speed measurements ranged from 2.25 to 3.66 m/s at the 12 o'clock position in the second patient. The bowel wall (*arrows*) of the second patient was circumferentially stiffened based on the color elastogram and was considerably stiffer and likely much more fibrotic than the first patient

Second, change in bowel wall stiffness over time may be able to assess the efficacy of medical therapy, document progression of bowel damage, and possibly predict a variety of important outcomes, such as the impending development of intestinal obstruction or penetrating complications, upcoming need for hospitalization or surgery, etc.

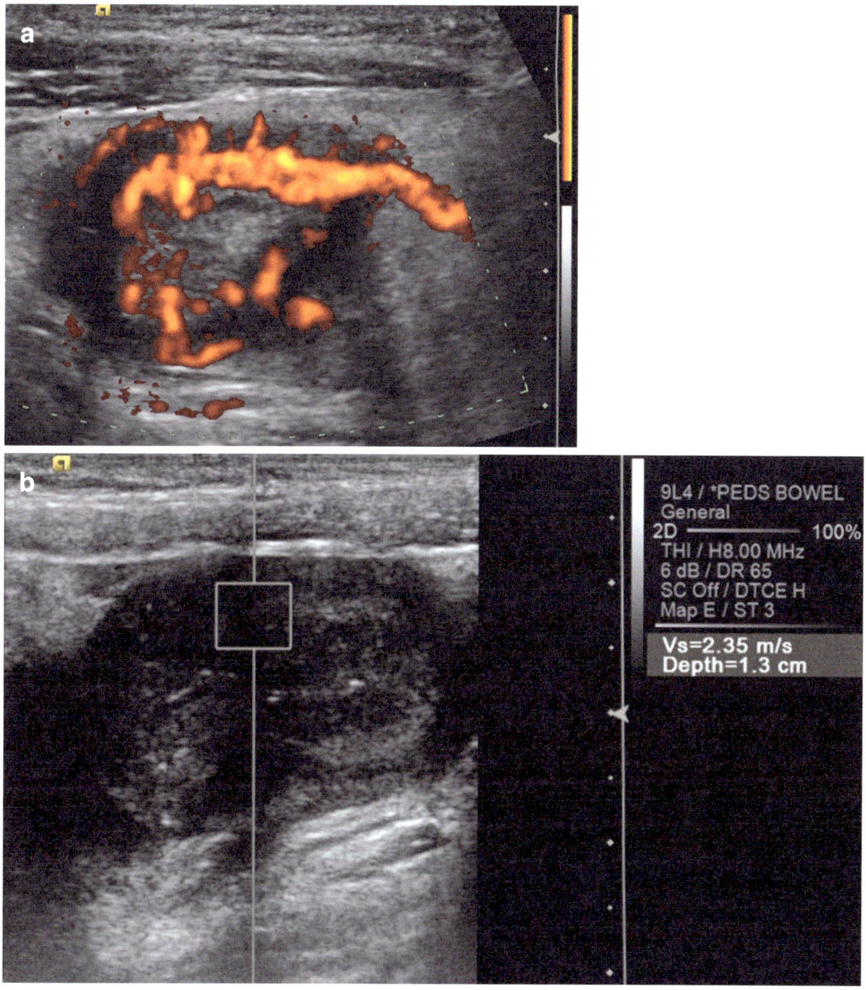

Fig. 3.7 Teenage boy with stricturing ileal small bowel Crohn's disease. (**a**) Power Doppler image in the region of the small bowel stricture shows markedly increased blood flow, indicative of substantial active inflammation. (**b**) Point shear wave speed measurement from the stricture measures 2.35 m/s, suggesting abnormal stiffening of the bowel wall and likely transmural fibrosis

3.5 Challenges and Obstacles

There remain multiple challenges and obstacles to the widespread adoption of using ultrasound elastographic methods to evaluate the bowel in Crohn's disease. Strain elastography remains primarily semiquantitative and quasi-static. The values obtained also are to some degree dependent on the transducer pressure (stress) applied by the operator. One potential method for making strain assessment of the bowel more quantitative and operator-independent (reproducible) is by assessing change in bowel wall deformation (bowel wall strain) with increasing ultrasound transducer pressure (increasing stress, measured as applied strain to the entire abdomen), so-called nonlinear strain elastography. Using the method described above by Xu et al. [17], developed bowel wall strain can be plotted as a function of applied abdominal strain, and a continuous nonlinear parameter can be derived. Currently available ultrasound systems assume that tissue strain increases linearly with increasing stress [13]. Research is ongoing in the area of nonlinear strain elastography.

The primary challenge for shear wave elastography of the bowel relates to performing this technique in a relatively small, tubular structure. While the single bowel wall thickness in Crohn's disease strictures is commonly 5–15 mm, the bowel is a cylindrical structure with a well-defined serosa. Based on this tissue geometry, shear waves may be subject to interaction with interfaces/boundaries, where the waves rebound off of interfaces and result in incorrect shear wave speed measurements [15]. The lack of established shear wave speed values for purely inflamed, purely fibrotic, and mixed inflammatory and fibrotic strictures is also a limitation, and these values may vary slightly based on the ultrasound system used as manufacturers have yet to standardize system design and settings (e.g., excitation frequency) [25].

Finally, both strain elastography and shear wave elastography have common limitations. Depth of bowel in the abdomen (distance from the abdominal wall) is a particular challenge to high-quality imaging that may prevent assessment of deep pelvic bowel loops or even evaluation of superficial bowel loops in overweight and obese patients. Also, both techniques assess tissue elasticity but fail to account for tissue viscosity [13]. However, despite these challenges, ultrasound elastography remains a promising imaging technique for characterizing thick-walled, often narrowed intestine in pediatric and adult Crohn's disease patients. The authors are optimistic about this imaging method as there is continuing research in this area, and there is a small but increasing body of published literature supporting its use in clinical practice.

References

1. Dillman JR, Smith EA, Sanchez RJ, et al. Pediatric small bowel Crohn disease: correlation of US and MR enterography. Radiographics. 2015;35(3):835–48.
2. Biko DM, Rosenbaum DG, Anupindi SA. Ultrasound features of pediatric Crohn disease: a guide for case interpretation. Pediatr Radiol. 2015;45(10):1557–66.
3. Dillman JR, Dehkordy SF, Smith EA, et al. Defining the ultrasound longitudinal natural history of newly diagnosed pediatric small bowel Crohn disease treated with infliximab and infliximab-azathioprine combination therapy. Pediatr Radiol. 2017;47(8):924–34.
4. Maconi G, Sampietro GM, Parente F, et al. Contrast radiology, computed tomography and ultrasonography in detecting internal fistulas and intra-abdominal abscesses in Crohn's disease: a prospective comparative study. Am J Gastroenterol. 2003;98(7):1545–55.
5. Bruining D, Zimmermann EM, Loftus EV Jr, et al. Consensus recommendations for evaluation, interpretation and utilization of CT and MR enterography in patients with small bowel Crohn's disease. Radiology. 2018;286(3):776–99.

6. Lu C, Gui X, Chen W, Fung T, Novak K, Wilson SR. Ultrasound shear wave elastography and contrast enhancement: effective biomarkers in Crohn's disease strictures. Inflamm Bowel Dis. 2017;23(3):421–30.
7. Adler J, Punglia DR, Dillman JR, et al. Computed tomography enterography findings correlate with tissue inflammation, not fibrosis in resected small bowel Crohn's disease. Inflamm Bowel Dis. 2012;18(5):849–56.
8. Barkmeier DT, Dillman JR, Al-Hawary M, et al. MR enterography-histology comparison in resected pediatric small bowel Crohn disease strictures: can imaging predict fibrosis? Pediatr Radiol. 2016;46(4):498–507.
9. Rimola J, Planell N, Rodríguez S, et al. Characterization of inflammation and fibrosis in Crohn's disease lesions by magnetic resonance imaging. Am J Gastroenterol. 2015;110(3):432–40.
10. Bettenworth D, Rieder F. Reversibility of stricturing Crohn's disease-fact or fiction? Inflamm Bowel Dis. 2016;22(1):241–7.
11. Malgras B, Pautrat K, Dray X, et al. Multidisciplinary management of gastrointestinal fibrotic stenosis in Crohn's disease. Dig Dis Sci. 2015;60(5):1152–68.
12. Ophir J, Céspedes I, Ponnekanti H, Yazdi Y, Li X. Elastography: a quantitative method for imaging the elasticity of biological tissues. Ultrason Imaging. 1991;13(2):111–34.
13. Sigrist RMS, Liau J, Kaffas AE, Chammas MC, Willmann JK. Ultrasound elastography: review of techniques and clinical applications. Theranostics. 2017;7(5):1303–29.
14. Sarvazyan AP, Rudenko OV, Swanson SD, Fowlkes JB, Emelianov SY. Shear wave elasticity imaging: a new ultrasonic technology of medical diagnostics. Ultrasound Med Biol. 1998;24(9):1419–35.
15. Nightingale K. Acoustic radiation force impulse (ARFI) imaging: a review. Curr Med Imaging Rev. 2011;7(4):328–39.
16. Kim K, Johnson LA, Jia C, et al. Noninvasive ultrasound elasticity imaging (UEI) of Crohn's disease: animal model. Ultrasound Med Biol. 2008;34(6):902–12.
17. Xu J, Tripathy S, Rubin JM, et al. A new nonlinear parameter in the developed strain-to-applied strain of the soft tissues and its application in ultrasound elasticity imaging. Ultrasound Med Biol. 2012;38(3):511–23.
18. Havre RF, Leh S, Gilja OH, et al. Strain assessment in surgically resected inflammatory and neoplastic bowel lesions. Ultraschall Med. 2014;35(2):149–58.
19. Baumgart DC, Müller HP, Grittner U, et al. US-based real-time elastography for the detection of fibrotic gut tissue in patients with stricturing Crohn disease. Radiology. 2015;275(3):889–99.
20. Fraquelli M, Branchi F, Cribiù FM, et al. The role of ultrasound elasticity imaging in predicting ileal fibrosis in Crohn's disease patients. Inflamm Bowel Dis. 2015;21(11):2605–12.
21. Pescatori LC, Mauri G, Savarino E, Pastorelli L, Vecchi M, Sconfienza LM. Bowel sonoelastography in patients with Crohn's disease: a systematic review. Ultrasound Med Biol. 2018;44(2):297–302.
22. Orlando S, Fraquelli M, Coletta M, et al. Ultrasound elasticity imaging predicts therapeutic outcomes of patients with Crohn's disease treated with anti-tumor necrosis factor antibodies. J Crohns Colitis. 2018;12(1):63–70.
23. Dillman JR, Stidham RW, Higgins PD, Moons DS, Johnson LA, Rubin JM. US elastography-derived shear wave velocity helps distinguish acutely inflamed from fibrotic bowel in a Crohn disease animal model. Radiology. 2013;267(3):757–66.
24. Dillman JR, Stidham RW, Higgins PD, et al. Ultrasound shear wave elastography helps discriminate low-grade from high-grade bowel wall fibrosis in ex vivo human intestinal specimens. J Ultrasound Med. 2014;33(12):2115–23.
25. Hall TJ, Milkowski A, Garra B, et al. RSNA/QIBA: shear wave speed as a biomarker for liver fibrosis staging. In: Ultrasonics symposium (IUS) IEEE international. New York: IEEE; 2013. p. 397–400.

MR and CT Imaging Techniques of the Bowel

4

Flavius F. Guglielmo, Christopher G. Roth, and Donald G. Mitchell

Abstract

MR and CT enterography play an integral role in managing patients with a variety of gastrointestinal conditions such as inflammatory bowel disease (IBD), non-IBD enteritis, small bowel and mesenteric masses, intermittent or low-grade small bowel obstruction, obscure gastrointestinal bleeding, and celiac disease. However, to facilitate optimal interpretation, high-quality state-of-the-art imaging is necessary. In this chapter, we provide a detailed review of the techniques for performing both MR and CT enterography. The authors have implemented these MR and CT protocols on a variety of MR and CT clinical scanners.

4.1 General Principles

4.1.1 Enterography Indications

In many centers, MR enterography (MRE) and CT enterography (CTE) have become the default small bowel imaging study essentially replacing traditional barium-based fluoroscopic exams (i.e., small bowel series and enteroclysis) [1, 2]. Indications for performing MRE or CTE are listed in Table 4.1 [1, 3–6]. While the indications have some overlap, the following principles should be considered when choosing between MRI and CT for small bowel imaging. Since MRE does not use ionizing radiation, this test is preferred for patients with Crohn's disease (CD) or polyposis syndromes as many of these patients present earlier in life and may

F. F. Guglielmo (✉) · C. G. Roth · D. G. Mitchell
Department of Radiology, Thomas Jefferson University, 132 South 10th Street, Philadelphia, 19107, PA, USA
e-mail: Flavius.Guglielmo@jefferson.edu; Christopher.Roth@jefferson.edu; Donald.Mitchell@jefferson.edu

J. Rimola (ed.), *Cross-Sectional Imaging in Crohn's Disease*,
https://doi.org/10.1007/978-3-319-96586-4_4

Table 4.1 Indications for MR and CT enterography

MR enterography	CT enterography
Diagnosis of IBD—evaluate disease activity and extent	Known Crohn's disease (not in the perioperative period)
Follow-up of IBD—disease activity and treatment response	Possible Crohn's disease or other causes of small bowel inflammation
Evaluation of IBD complications (e.g., stricture, fistula, or abscess)	Obscure gastrointestinal bleeding
Small bowel masses including polyposis syndromes	Chronic diarrhea and/or abdominal pain
Intermittent or low-grade small bowel obstruction	Chronic mesenteric ischemia
Celiac disease	Celiac disease
Non-IBD enteritis (e.g., infection, vasculitis, treatment-related enteritis)	

IBD, inflammatory bowel disease

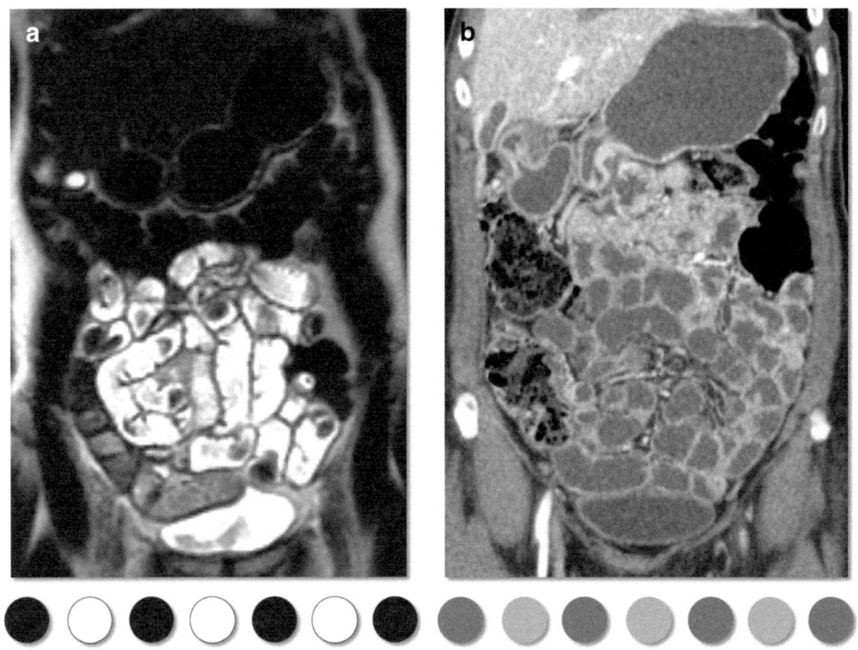

Fig. 4.1 Coronal heavily T2-weighted image (**a**) and coronal CT enterography image (**b**). With MRI, the difference in signal intensity between the fluid in the lumen and bowel wall is greater than the density difference on CT which can increase the conspicuity of bowel abnormalities compared to CT

require multiple imaging studies for many years [1, 3, 7–9]. In Crohn's disease, MRI has an additional advantage over CT due to higher contrast resolution, making MRI more sensitive for identifying bowel wall edema and fibrosis (Fig. 4.1). Also, perianal fistulas, which occur in up to 25% of CD patients, are more readily identified with MRI than with CT. Finally, for all patients, compared to static CT images, MRE adds another dimension to small bowel imaging when "cine MRE" is performed providing small bowel peristalsis evaluation to help identify bowel strictures, adhesions, and small bowel masses [10]. On the other hand, due to the higher spatial resolution and faster image acquisition time, CT is the test of choice for patients with obscure gastrointestinal bleeding, subtle small bowel masses, or difficulty with breath holding [10].

4.1.2 Enteric Contrast Agents

With both MR and CT enterography, the goal of administering enteric contrast agents is to adequately distend the small bowel and provide homogeneous opacification of the lumen with high contrast between the lumen and bowel wall while having no serious adverse side effects [6]. The most commonly used MR enteric agents are "biphasic" agents which have low signal intensity on T1-weighted images and high signal intensity on T2-weighted images (Fig. 4.2) [11–14]. Biphasic agents include low-density barium sulfate suspension (Volumen, Bracco Diagnostics, Princeton, New Jersey), mannitol, sorbitol, polyethylene glycol, water (only effective for stomach and duodenum due to rapid absorption from the small bowel), methylcellulose, and locust bean gum [12, 15–18]. These same contrast agents are used for CT enterography due to the relative low density of the contrast agents which allows identification of bowel wall and mucosal enhancement which can be obscured when standard barium or iodine solutions are used (Fig. 4.3) [19, 20].

The choice of enteric contrast agent depends on patient tolerance and regional availability. A study by Young et al. [21] compared four different biphasic agents

Enteric Contrast Agents	T1 Weighted Signal Intensity	T2 Weighted Signal Intensity	Examples
Biphasic	●	○	Low density barium sulfate suspension Mannitol Sorbitol Polyethylene glycol Water Methylcellulose Locust bean gum
Negative	●	●	Ferumoxsil oral suspension Oral superparamagnetic particles Perfluoroctylbromide
Positive	○	○	Diluted gadolinium Fruit juices containing manganese (e.g. grapefruit, pineapple, or blueberry juice) * Milk with a high fat content

***Note:** Fruit juices may act as negative oral contrast agents if the manganese concentrations are very high.

Fig. 4.2 The signal intensities of the different MRI enteric contrast agents on T1-weighted and T2-weighted images

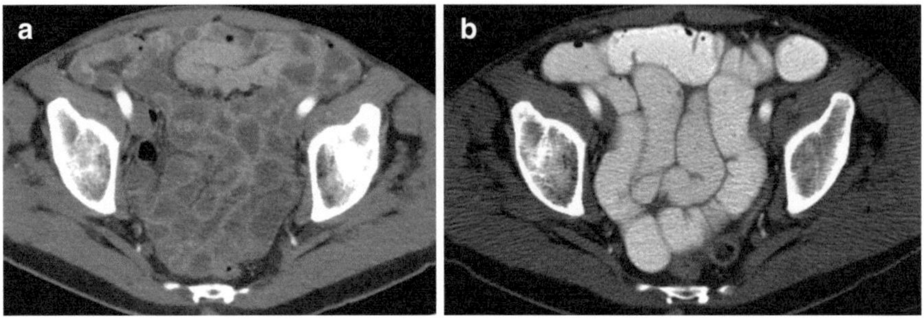

Fig. 4.3 CT enterogram using low-density barium sulfate suspension (**a**) and standard barium solution (**b**). In image (**a**), mural and mucosal enhancement is readily identifiable with neutral oral contrast while much less conspicuous in image (**b**) due to the positive oral contrast

and found that low-density barium sulfate suspension and polyethylene glycol had better bowel distension than water or methylcellulose. However, polyethylene glycol was the most difficult to drink and was the agent patients least preferred to drink. In the United States, low-density barium sulfate suspension is commonly chosen for both MR and CT enterography protocols, which is the case in our practice. An alternative is a newer commercially available contrast agent containing a thickening agent (Breeza for neutral abdominopelvic imaging, Beekley Medical) which has been shown to have similar side effects and equivalent small bowel distention compared to a low-density barium sulfate suspension although was rated higher by patients in taste and willingness to repeat the drinking protocol for subsequent exams [22]. In countries where these agents are not available, polyethylene glycol, methylcellulose, or a solution combined with sorbitol, mannitol, or locust bean gum can be used [6, 15, 18, 23]. Finally, milk can be a cost-effective option for CT enterography [24].

As a general rule, the patient should drink as much enteric contrast as possible (i.e., 1350–1500 mL) without the agent passing through the patient during the exam [2, 25]. For low-density barium suspension, one bottle of 450 ml is administered every 20 min for a total of three bottles. If needed, an additional 250–500 mL of water can be administered right before imaging for better distension of the stomach and proximal small bowel while reducing the amount of administered hyperosmolar fluid [2, 26].

4.1.3 Intravenous Contrast Material

With both MR and CT enterography, intravenous contrast administration is needed to identify abnormal enhancement of the bowel wall and mucosa, inflammatory masses, and the walls of infected fluid collections, perienteric fistulas, and sinus tracts. For MR enterography, an extracellular space contrast agent (ECSA) is the agent of choice. In our practice, we prefer to use the ECSA gadobenate dimeglumine because of the stronger enhancement due to higher relaxivity compared to other ECSAs. For patients that have had multiple MRE exams perform, a macrocyclic agent can be used such as gadoterate meglumine, gadobutrol, or gadoteridol because of the higher stability compared to linear agents [27, 28] (Table 4.2). For all ECSAs, a standard dose of 0.1 mmol/kg is administered at 2 mL/s followed by a saline flush.

For CT enterography, most centers use iodinated contrast containing 300 mg/mL of iodine, and 100–150 mL of contrast media is injected. Contrast is generally injected at a rate of 3–4 mL/s. For patients that cannot receive iodinated contrast due to a severe contrast allergy or chronic renal disease, MR enterography is the preferred option. For patients that cannot receive gadolinium due to severe chronic renal disease, noncontrast MR enterography that includes diffusion-weighted and T2-weighted images is an acceptable alternative. Finally, for patients in which MRI is contraindicated or cannot be performed due to claustrophobia, a noncontrast CT enterography or enteroclysis using positive enteric contrast agents or a standard small bowel series or small bowel enteroclysis can be performed [29].

For CTE, scanning can be performed during the "enteric" phase (50 s after injection) or the portal venous phase (60–70 s after injection) [27, 30–33]. For MRE, multiphase dynamic post-contrast 3D fat-suppressed gradient-echo images can be obtained including precontrast, late arterial phase (30–35 s after injection), and portal venous phase sequences. While maximum small bowel enhancement occurs during the enteric phase, a study by Vandenbroucke et al. showed that there was no significant difference in Crohn's disease lesion detection between the enteric and portal venous phases [34]. Finally, with MRI, studies have shown that delayed imaging up to 8 min after injection can improve lesion detection and grading disease activity with Crohn's disease [35, 36].

There are two potential pitfalls to be aware of when interpreting MRE and CTE exams. First, CT attenuation (and signal intensity on post-contrast T1-weighted images) is normally greater in the jejunum than in the ileum and is greater in collapsed small bowel segments compared to distended small bowel segments (Fig. 4.4) [29, 37–39]. Thus, when interpreting MRE or CTE exams, it is important to compare CT attenuation and post-contrast T1 signal intensity of jejunal small bowel segments to other jejunal segments and ileal segments to other ileal segments. Also, on MRE, the same bowel segment should be evaluated on multiple pulse sequences to determine if a bowel segment is truly abnormal or just transiently collapsed and normal. This is one of the advantages of MRE compared to CTE which usually has only one phase compared to the multiple sequences in an MRE exam.

4.1.4 Antiperistaltic Agents

With MR enterography, small bowel peristalsis limits bowel wall evaluation due to blurring from motion artifact. This is predominantly an issue with 3D gradient-echo (GRE) sequences which generally have a relatively long acquisition time of 15–19 s. While several studies [40, 41] reported similar accuracy when interpreting MR enterography exams without using antiperistaltic agents, most academic centers

Table 4.2 The seven commercially available extracellular space gadolinium-based contrast agents

Generic name	Product or trade name	Structure	Ionicity	T1 relaxivity at 1.5 T	Hepatobiliary excretion	Concentration (mmol/mL)	Recommended dosage (mmol/kg)
Gadoterate meglumine	Dotarem	Macrocyclic	Ionic	3.4–3.8	0	0.5	0.1
Gadobutrol	Gadavist/ Gadovist	Macrocyclic	Nonionic	4.9–5.5	0	1	0.1
Gadoteridol	ProHance	Macrocyclic	Nonionic	3.9–4.3	0	0.5	0.1
Gadopentetate dimeglumine	Magnevist	Linear	Ionic	3.9–4.3	0	0.5	0.1
Gadoversetamide	Optimark	Linear	Nonionic	4.4–5	0	0.5	0.1
Gadodiamide	Omniscan	Linear	Nonionic	4–4.6	0	0.5	0.1
Gadobenate dimeglumine	MultiHance	Linear	Ionic	6–6.6	3–5%	0.5	0.1

Modified with permission from Ref. [21], Copyright Springer Science+Business Media New York 2016

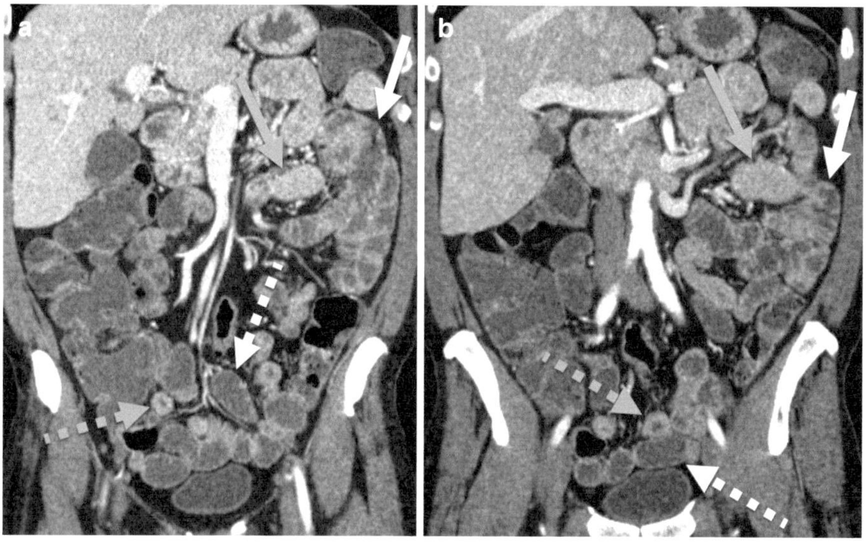

Fig. 4.4 Normal CT enterogram using low-density barium sulfate suspension (**a**) and (**b**). Collapsed loops of jejunum (*solid gray arrows*) have higher attenuation than distended loops of jejunum (*solid white arrows*), and collapsed loops of ileum (*dashed gray arrows*) have higher attenuation than distended loops of ileum (solid dashed arrows). Also, overall attenuation of the jejunum is greater than the ileum

now routinely administer these agents to improve image quality and facilitate exam interpretation. In a paper by Ziech et al., 24 academic radiologists were surveyed. They found that 92% used antiperistaltic agents including hyoscine butylbromide (Buscopan; Boehringer Ingelheim, Ingelheim Germany) in 82% and glucagon (Glucagen; Novo Nordisk, Bagsvaerd, Denmark) in 18% [42].

In the United States, the most commonly used antiperistaltic agent is glucagon which is administered at a dose of 0.5–1 mg and usually given intravenously immediately before obtaining the pre- and post-gadolinium 3D GRE series [43]. In some centers, a split dose is given, with part of the dose given before the T2-weighted sequences and the remainder before the pre- and post-gadolinium 3D GRE series. Glucagon can also be given intramuscularly, although the onset of antiperistaltic effect will be slower [44]. The most common side effects with glucagon are nausea and vomiting which can occur up to 3 h after injecting. Injecting slowly (i.e., over a 5-min period) has been shown to reduce side effects [38].

Hyoscine butylbromide (Buscopan) is the most commonly administered antiperistaltic agent outside of the United States. The dose is 20 mg which is administered intravenously as a single or split dose using two [12] or three [45, 46] different injections. Similar to glucagon, hyoscine butylbromide can be given intramuscularly although with a slower onset of antiperistaltic action [44]. Hyoscine butylbromide is not available to use in the United States.

Newer 3D GRE sequences are now available which have shorter acquisition times that can lead to less motion artifact from bowel peristalsis. Finally, antiperistaltic administration is less important when performing CT enterography due to CT's rapid acquisition time.

4.2 MR Enterography

4.2.1 Patient Preparation

With MR enterography (MRE), patients should ideally fast beginning 4–6 h before the exam. This prevents bladder overfilling during the study and leaves the stomach empty, so the patient can drink the maximum amount of enteric contrast [47]. Beginning 1 h before the exam, the patient begins drinking enteric contrast such as one bottle (450 mL) of low-density barium sulfate suspension (Volumen, Bracco Diagnostics, Princeton, NJ) every 20 min for a total of three bottles (1350 mL). If possible, patients are scanned in the prone position which helps improve small bowel distension and separation, decreases motion artifact, and reduces the volume to scan [11]. If patients cannot be scanned prone, supine positioning is usually sufficient. One paper by Cronin et al. [48] showed that there was no difference in lesion detection between supine and prone positioning. A standard intravenous dose of an extracellular space gadolinium-based contrast agent is administered. In our practice, we prefer 0.1 mmol/kg of gadobenate dimeglumine (MultiHance, Bracco Diagnostics, Princeton, NJ) due to the higher relaxivity compared to other extracellular space contrast agents (Table 4.2) [27, 28, 49]. Finally, an antiperistaltic agent should be administered to decrease small bowel peristalsis.

4.2.2 MR Enterography Technical Considerations

To achieve the best image quality, MR enterography should ideally be performed on a high-field MR system with a field strength of 1.5 T or greater. A phased array coil or combination of phased array coils should be used to ensure complete coverage of the bowel in the abdomen and pelvis [3, 4, 50]. Using a 3 T MRI can improve the signal-to-noise ratio and spatial resolution of the exam but may be limited by higher specific absorption rates and imaging artifacts such as dielectric effects [6, 51].

4.2.3 MR Enterography Protocol

Thorough evaluation of the bowel with MRI is possible by performing an MR enterography protocol like the one in Table 4.3 [2, 52]. After obtaining a three-plane localizer series, a three-plane balanced steady-state free precession series (BSSFP) followed by axial and coronal heavily T2-weighted sequences and axial or coronal 2D dual gradient-echo in- and out-of-phase series are obtained. In most centers, intravenous glucagon or Buscopan is then administered followed by coronal dynamic pre- and post-gadolinium-enhanced fat-suppressed 3D gradient-echo pulse

Table 4.3 MR enterography pulse sequences and parameters (1.5 T)

Sequence	Plane	FOV	Matrix	Slice thickness/ gap (mm)	TR (ms)	TE (ms)	Flip angle	Fat suppression
SSFSE survey (localizer series)[a]	Three-plane	45	320 × 192	8/0	Min	80	90	No
BSSFP	Three-plane	38	192 × 288	5/0	Min	Min	60	No
SSFSE (heavily T2W)	Coronal	42	256 × 192	5/0	Min	180	90	No
SSFSE (heavily T2W)	Axial	38	256 × 192	5/0	Min	180	90	No
2D dual gradient echo in- and out-of-phase[b]	Axial	38	256 × 192	7/0.5	265	2.1/4.4	90	No
Dynamic multiphase fat-suppressed 3D GRE (pre, late arterial, and portal venous phase)[c]	Coronal	42	320 × 224	4.4/2.2	Min	Min	12	Yes
Moderately T2W FS	Coronal	44	256 × 224	5/0	700	80	90	Yes
Moderately T2W FS	Axial	38	256 × 224	5/0	700	80	90	Yes
T1-weighted 3D spoiled GRE (delayed phase)	Coronal	42	320 × 224	4.4/2.2	Min	Min	12	Yes
T1-weighted 3D spoiled GRE (delayed phase)	Axial	40	256 × 192	4.4/2.2	Min	Min	12	Yes
Cine BSSFP[d]	Coronal	40	224 × 288	8/1.5	3.8	1.7	70	No
Diffusion-weighted images	Axial	36	128 × 128	6/1	7000	73	90	Yes

Modified with permission from Ref. [21], Copyright Springer Science+Business Media New York 2016

2D two-dimensional, *3D* three-dimensional, *BSSFP* balanced steady-state free precession, *FOV* field of view, *FS* fat suppression, *GRE* gradient echo, *mm* millimeters, *ms* milliseconds, *SSFSE* single-shot fast spin echo, *T2W* T2 weighted, *TE* echo time, *TR* repetition time

[a]T1 weighted or balanced steady-state free precession sequences can be performed instead

[b]The 2D dual gradient-echo in- and out-of-phase series is a 2D acquisition. On more modern MR equipment, a two-point Dixon 3D acquisition is obtained which has parameters that match the pre- and post-gadolinium fat-suppressed 3D GRE series "water" image (except for the echo time)

[c]Antiperistaltic agents are usually administered before this sequence. In some centers, a split dose is given, with part of the dose given before the T2-weighted sequences and the remainder before the dynamic multiphase 3D GRE series

[d]Cine BSSFP series should be performed before administering antiperistaltic agents or any time during the protocol if antiperistaltic agents are not administered. Parameters for the cine BSSFP series are variable for different MR vendors. General Electric parameters are displayed

sequences (FS 3DGRE). Next, coronal and axial fat-suppressed moderately T2 weighted, coronal and axial delayed post-contrast FS 3DGRE, and axial diffusion-weighted sequences are obtained. A coronal cine BSSFP series can be obtained at the beginning of the study if antiperistaltics are administered or anytime during the study if they are not.

The MRE protocol in Table 4.3 takes about 45 min to complete. In the sections that follow below, each pulse sequence will be covered with a discussion about the clinical utility, advantages, and disadvantages.

4.2.4 Localizer Series

The localizer series is usually a rapid sequence obtained with a moderately large field of view in three planes (i.e., axial, sagittal, and coronal). Several pulse sequences can be used including single-shot fast spin echo, T1-weighted, or balanced steady-state free precession sequences. The default imaging technique set by MR vendors usually includes thick slices (e.g., 10 mm) with significant gaps between slices (e.g., 5 mm). However, this can be changed to thinner slices and gaps (e.g., 6 mm/1 mm) to improve the diagnostic utility of this series.

4.2.4.1 Clinical Utility

The localizer series is performed to confirm that the torso array coil is positioned so that the abdomen and pelvis is included within the sensitive volume of the coil.

4.2.4.2 Advantages

For case interpretation, this is generally the only series in an MRE protocol that is obtained in the sagittal plane and may be the best imaging plane to identify spine compression fractures or localizing spine lesions [27].

4.2.4.3 Disadvantages

If this series includes thick slices with large gaps between slices (e.g., 10/5 mm), misregistration artifact can be a significant problem.

4.2.5 Balanced Steady-State Free Precession (BSSFP)

BSSFP is a bright-blood technique in which all three gradients (i.e., frequency, phase, and slice) are refocused and magnetization is continually preserved rather than spoiled [53, 54]. This sequence is very useful as a three-plane localizer series but can also be performed as a stand-alone axial or coronal series. Examples of vendor names for BSSFP sequences include balanced fast-field echo (BFFE), true fast imaging with steady-state precession (true FISP), and fast imaging employing steady-state acquisition (FIESTA) (Figs. 4.5 and 4.6).

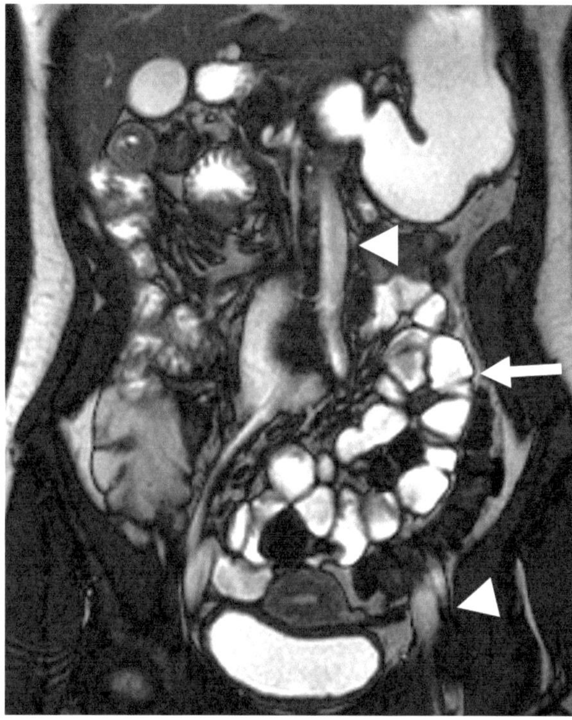

Fig. 4.5 Coronal balanced steady-state free precession image (BSSFP). With BSSFP, fluid (*arrow*) and blood vessels such as the aorta (*arrowheads*) both have high signal intensity. For this reason, this "white blood" technique can confirm patency of blood vessels

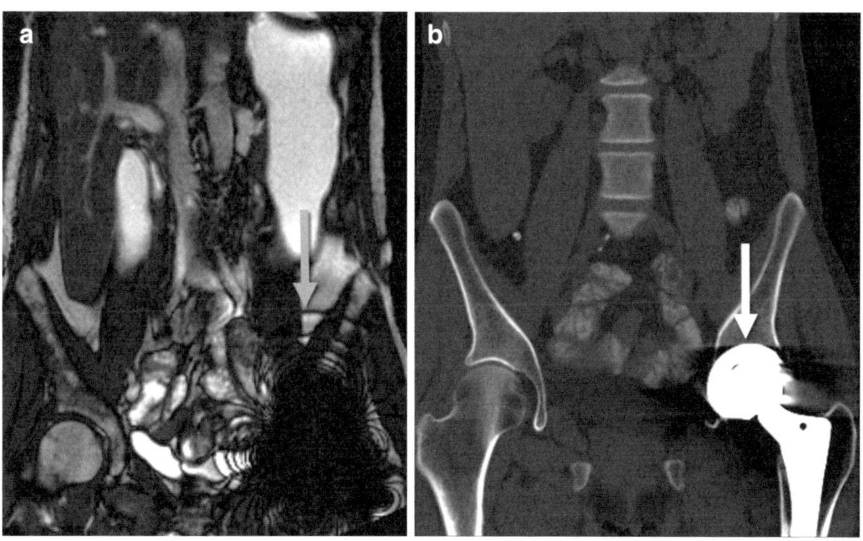

Fig. 4.6 Coronal balanced steady-state free precession image (BSSFP) (**a**) and corresponding coronal CT image (**b**). There is significant susceptibility artifact (gray arrow in **a**) due to a metallic left hip prosthesis which is demonstrated on CT (white arrow in **b**)

4.2.5.1 Clinical Utility

BSSFP sequences can be used to evaluate the overall small bowel for abnormalities such as dilatation or wall thickening. The high signal intensity of blood vessels is useful for evaluating the abdominal vasculature for patency (Fig. 4.5).

4.2.5.2 Advantages

BSSFP sequences are the most motion resistance series in an MRE protocol. This can be helpful for patients that have difficulty holding their breath. Also, the bright-blood technique can help evaluate blood vessel patency in cases where gadolinium cannot be administered.

4.2.5.3 Disadvantages

Due to chemical shift artifact, on sequences that are not fat-suppressed, a "black boundary" artifact occurs at the periphery of the bowel wall which precludes precise measurement of the bowel wall for thickening [15]. Also, due to the lack of refocusing pulses, significant susceptibility artifact can occur due to bowel gas or metallic structures which can limit evaluation of a portion of the abdomen (Fig. 4.6) [55]. Finally, the high signal intensity of both blood vessels and cysts or ducts can cause confusion differentiating these structures [27].

4.2.6 Cine Balanced Steady-State Free Precession (Cine BSSFP)

Cine BSSFP is a bright-blood technique based on the same pulse sequences as the static BSSFP sequences (i.e., BFFE, true FISP, or FIESTA). However, at each imaging slice, multiple sequential phases are obtained and displayed sequentially to create a video depicting bowel peristalsis. Typically, between 10 and 20 slices are obtained with 25 phases per slice. A 12-slice cine BSSFP sequence takes about 4 min to complete. This series can be obtained without or with fat suppression (Fig. 4.7). Since this sequence evaluates small bowel peristalsis, this series must be performed before antiperistaltic agents are administered [15, 56].

4.2.6.1 Clinical Utility

Cine BSSFP sequences can be used to evaluate the overall small bowel for an increase in peristalsis (e.g., small bowel obstruction) or a decrease in peristalsis (e.g., ileus) or individual small bowel segments for relatively decreased peristalsis (e.g., bowel inflammation, stricture, or mass) [8, 9, 52, 57–61].

When interpreting cine BSSFP sequences, it is important to choose a frame rate on PACS which allows temporal separation of small bowel segments. At our institution, we have found that 12 frames per second is a good starting point. This frame rate can be increased or decreased depending on the speed of small bowel peristalsis. After setting the frame rate, the overall small bowel and individual small bowel segments are evaluated for a relative increase or decrease in peristalsis rate. Since there are no standards for peristalsis evaluation, identifying abnormal peristalsis is subjective and requires experience to develop an understanding of "normal" peristalsis first [56].

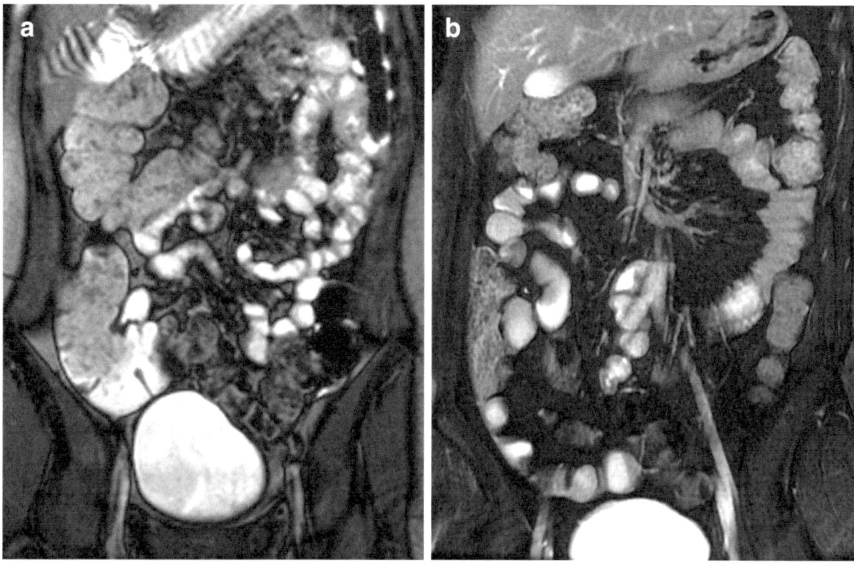

Fig. 4.7 Coronal cine balanced steady-state free precession image series in two different patients without (**a**) and with (**b**) fat suppression. The cine series in image (**a**) had 12 slices with 25 phases per slice, and the cine series in image (**b**) had 15 slices with 25 phases per slice

4.2.6.2 Advantages and Disadvantages

The same advantages and disadvantages of static BSSFP sequences pertain to cine BSSFP sequences.

4.2.7 T2-Weighted Sequences

For MRE studies, at our institution, we obtain two complementary T2-weighted sequences (T2WI), both using single-shot fast spin echo (SSFSE) technique because of its relative insensitivity to patient motion. This includes a "heavily T2-weighted" series with an effective echo time of 180–200 ms (Fig. 4.8) and a fat-suppressed "moderately T2-weighted" series with an effective echo time of 80–100 ms (Fig. 4.9) [27, 62, 63]. Heavily T2WI are ideally performed without fat suppression to improve delineation of organ boundaries and performed before gadolinium administration to avoid gadolinium's T2 shortening effects which can darken the renal collecting systems and liver hemangiomas [27]. Moderately T2WI can be performed post-gadolinium and with fat suppression, to improve the conspicuity of bowel wall edema, lymph nodes, and solid organ lesions [27, 63].

4.2.7.1 Clinical Utility

T2-weighted images are "fluid-sensitive" sequences and are the best sequence to evaluate for fluid collections, mural and perienteric edema, and fluid within fistulas

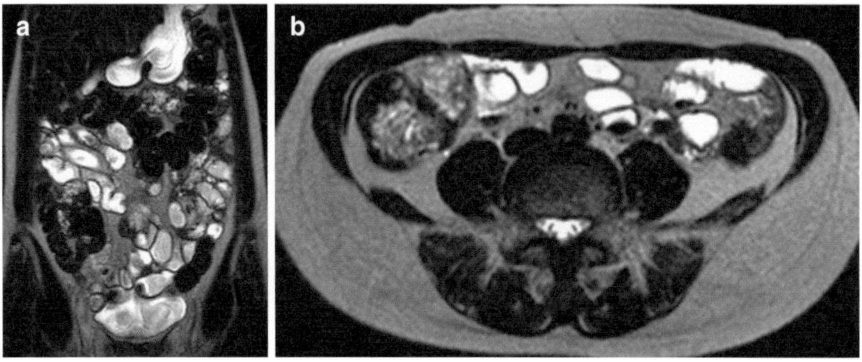

Fig. 4.8 Coronal (**a**) and axial (**b**) heavily T2-weighted images obtained with an effective echo time of 200 ms. This series is ideally performed before gadolinium administration and without fat suppression

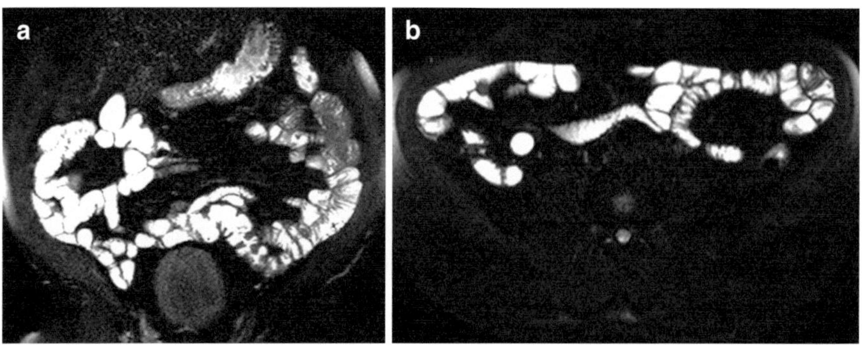

Fig. 4.9 Coronal (**a**) and axial (**b**) fat-suppressed moderately T2-weighted images obtained with an effective echo time of 80 ms. This series is ideally performed after gadolinium administration

and sinus tracts. T2WI can be used to measure bowel wall thickness to evaluate for thickening while also demonstrating mural edema, indicating active inflammation, and/or mural fibrosis [8, 9, 64].

4.2.7.2 Advantages

The multiple 180° refocusing pulses used to obtain T2W images result in less susceptibility artifact compared to all other series in the MRE protocol. Thus, metal clips or bowel gas will cause less distortion and blooming artifact, particularly on images without fat suppression.

4.2.7.3 Disadvantages

Intraluminal motion due to bowel peristalsis leads to "flow void" artifacts within bowel segments, likely due to saturation effects of fluid, which can simulate true intraluminal filling defects [15]. The way to mitigate this artifact is to evaluate the

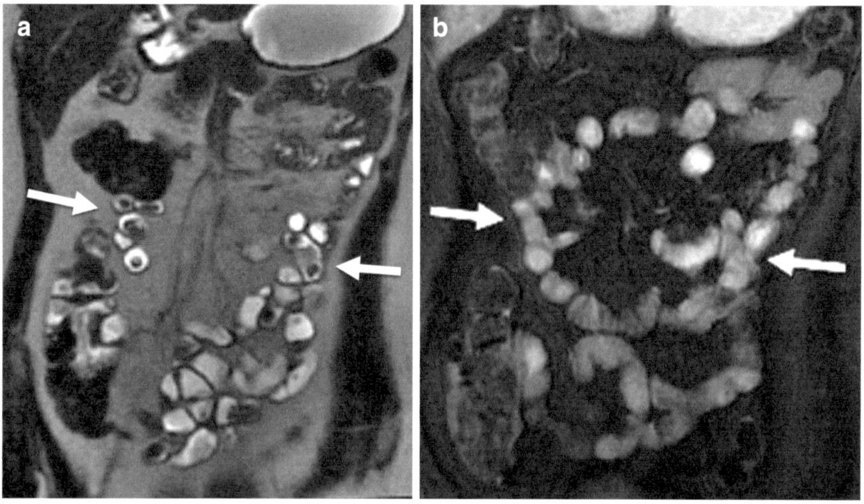

Fig. 4.10 Coronal heavily T2-weighted image with an effective echo time of 180 ms (**a**) and corresponding coronal cine balanced steady-state free precession (BSSFP) image (**b**). In the T2-weighted image, the round filling defects in the small bowel lumen (arrows in **a**) are flow void artifacts created by peristalsis. This is confirmed by correlating with the BSSFP series which has a faster acquisition time and does not show these filling defects (arrows in **b**)

corresponding BSSFP series which is not as prone to saturation effects (Fig. 4.10). Another limitation is a relatively low signal-to-noise ratio due to the single-shot acquisition technique, especially for fat-suppressed T2-weighted sequences.

4.2.8 Dual Gradient-Echo In- and Out-of-Phase

This is a gradient-echo (GRE) sequence in which two different echo times are obtained that optimize the precessional frequency difference between water and fat. At specific echo times proportional to the magnetic field strength, fat and water signal will be either in-phase or out-of-phase [65]. High signal occurs when water and fat signal are summed on in-phase images. The opposite occurs on out-of-phase images in which the sum of water and fat signal leads to decreased signal intensity (i.e., phase cancellation) [65, 66]. For older MR systems, this series is performed as a stand-alone 2D sequence. On more modern MR systems, this series is automatically obtained using a modified two-point Dixon fat-water separation technique to generate fat-suppressed 3D gradient-echo sequences [67, 68]. The advantage of this latter technique is thinner slices (e.g., 4 mm versus 7 mm) which match the fat-suppressed 3D gradient-echo images (i.e., "water image") and obtaining one less series which decreases total exam time. This series must be performed before gadolinium administration for optimal tissue characterization. Images can be obtained in either the coronal (Fig. 4.11) or axial plane.

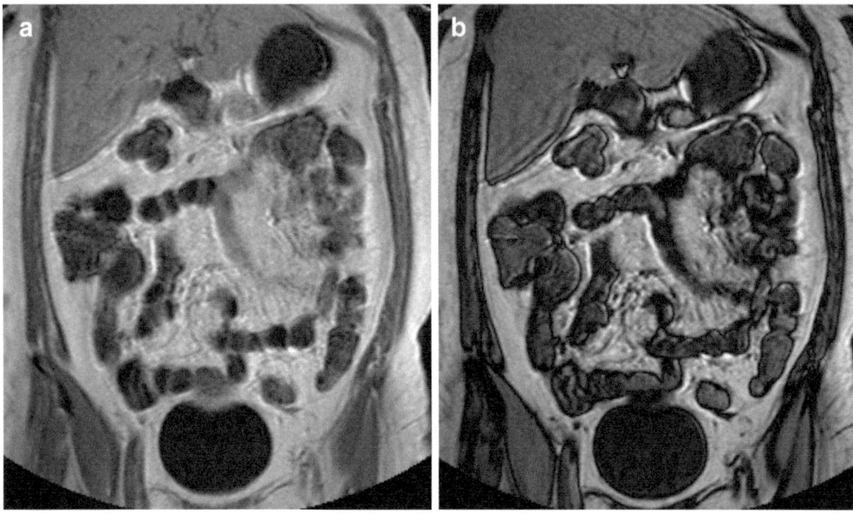

Fig. 4.11 Coronal in-phase (**a**) and out-of-phase (**b**) 2D gradient-echo images with an echo time (TE) of 4.6 and 2.3 ms, respectively

4.2.8.1 Clinical Utility

The dual gradient-echo in- and out-of-phase series provides T1-weighted information complementing the information provided by the fat-suppressed (T1 weighted) 3D GRE series. For example, when fat is present in the bowel wall which may indicate changes of long-standing inflammatory bowel disease, the wall will be hyperintense on in- and out-of-phase images and hypointense on fat-suppressed 3D GRE images. This series is also beneficial in characterizing findings incidentally found on MRE studies such as a fatty liver, liver or splenic iron overload, ovarian dermoids, or endometriosis [65, 66]. Finally, "blooming" of air bubbles within stool on in-phase images can help distinguish large bowel from small bowel.

4.2.8.2 Advantages

This is the only nonfat-suppressed T1-weighted sequence which when combined with other pulse sequences facilitates tissue characterization.

4.2.8.3 Disadvantages

Both 3D and 2D dual GRE sequences can be degraded by motion artifact created by bowel peristalsis due to a relatively long series acquisition duration.

4.2.9 Dynamic Multiphase Fat-Suppressed 3D Gradient Echo (3D GRE)

T1-weighted dynamic multiphase fat-suppressed 3D gradient-echo sequences are the "workhorse" sequence in a MRE exam, many times providing valuable information about the presence of bowel inflammation or fibrosis [26, 69]. To obtain this series, a volume of the abdomen is obtained with a single 15–19 s breath hold.

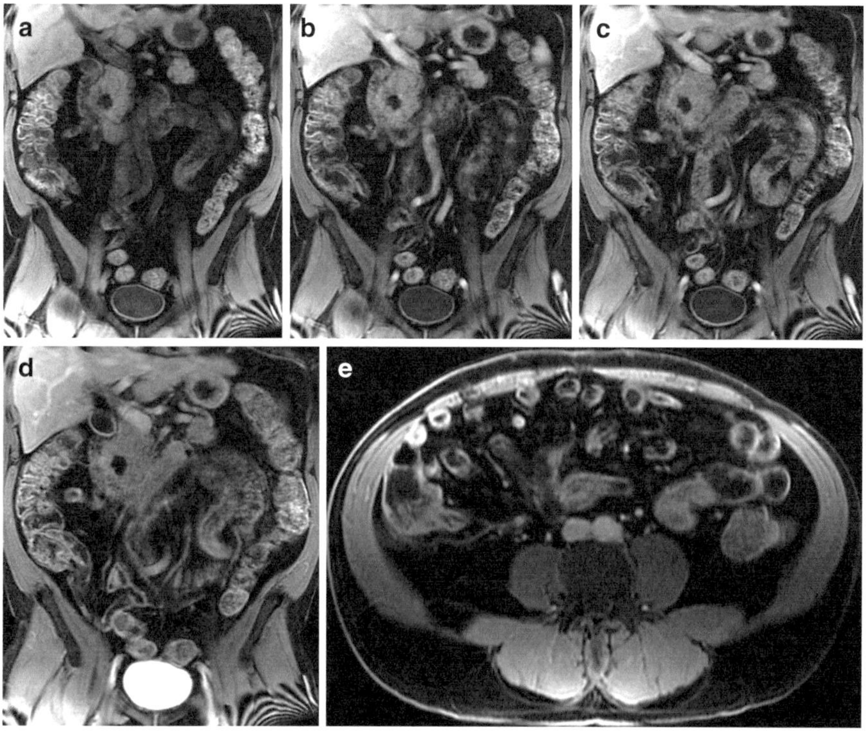

Fig. 4.12 Coronal precontrast (**a**), late arterial phase (**b**), and portal venous phase (**c**) contrast-enhanced 3D gradient-echo (GRE) images and delayed coronal (**d**) and axial 3D GRE images (**e**)

Precontrast and dynamic coronal late arterial and portal venous phase images are obtained followed by delayed phase coronal and axial images (Fig. 4.12). Given this series' relatively long acquisition duration, controlling small bowel peristalsis with antiperistaltic agents (discussed above) is especially important with 3D GRE [7]. However, newer 3D techniques with faster acquisition time and higher temporal resolution may decrease the motion sensitivity of this sequence.

Examples of vendor names for 3D GRE sequences include liver acquisition with volume acceleration (LAVA), T1 high-resolution isotropic volume excitation (THRIVE), and volumetric interpolated breath-hold examination (VIBE). Acronyms for more modern MRI systems that use the modified two-point Dixon technique for fat suppression include liver acquisition with volume acceleration-flexible (LAVA-Flex), modified Dixon (mDixon), and Dixon volumetric interpolated breath-hold examination (Dixon-VIBE).

4.2.9.1 Clinical Utility

This series is used to evaluate bowel wall thickness and the amount, pattern, and timing of bowel wall enhancement. Enhancement of non-bowel structures is also evaluated including lymph nodes and the walls of fluid collections, fistulas, and sinus tracts.

4.2.9.2 Advantages

The thin slice thickness (5 mm or less) and 50% overlap of the 3D GRE series allow better bowel tracking when scrolling through images on PACS compared to the other series in an MRE protocol, most of which are 2D acquisitions.

4.2.9.3 Disadvantages

Bowel wall blurring is a significant problem with this series, especially if antiperistaltics are not administered. Fortunately, many times bowel peristalsis is decreased in abnormal small bowel segments due to inflammation or stricturing, resulting in less motion artifact [40, 41, 52].

4.2.10 Diffusion-Weighted Images

Diffusion-weighted images (DWI) evaluate for water mobility within tissues. Tissues with either tense edema or dense cellularity will have high signal intensity on DWI. Typically, multiple b-values are obtained such as b-values of 0, 20, and 800. A b-value of 0 has no diffusion weighting. A b-value of 20 has minimal diffusion weighting which results in signal loss in blood vessels making tumors, edema, and fluid more conspicuous. A high b-value of 800–1000 negates signal intensity from fluid and normal bowel mucosa and is best for identifying inflammation [45, 70, 71]. When at least two b-values are obtained, an ADC map can be generated (Fig. 4.13). Tissues with abundant diffusion will display as high signal intensity on

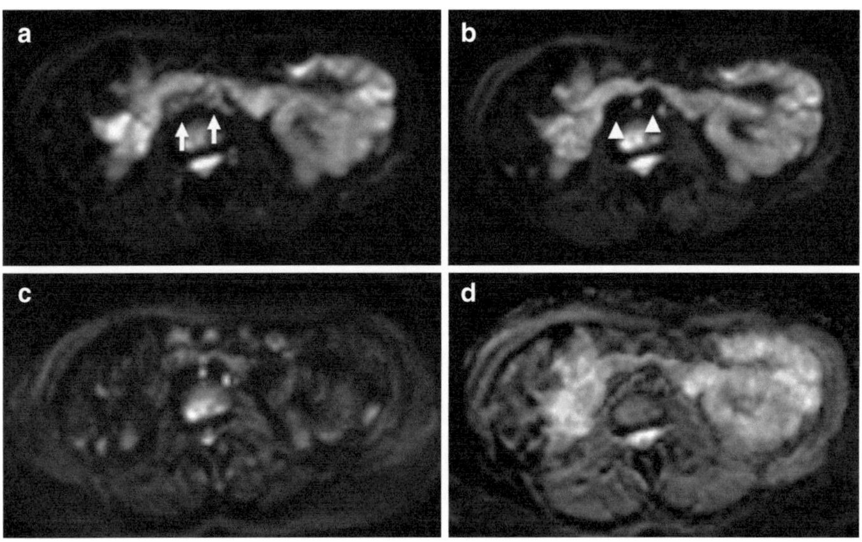

Fig. 4.13 Axial diffusion-weighted images with b-values of 0 (**a**), 20 (**b**), and 800 (**c**). With a b-value of 0, most blood vessels have high signal intensity (arrows in **a**), while with a b-value of 20, most blood vessels have dark signal intensity (arrowheads in **b**). When more than one b-value is obtained, an ADC map can be generated (**d**) to evaluate for restricted diffusion versus T2 shine through

the ADC map due to "T2 shine through." True restricted diffusion will display as low signal intensity on the ADC map [72, 73].

There are three methods for performing DWI including breath hold, respiratory triggered, and free breathing with multiple averages (e.g., 4–10). The latter two techniques take 3–6 min to complete. Free breathing has the highest signal-to-noise ratio and the most consistent suppression of respiratory motion, being less dependent on patient and operator variability [45, 74].

4.2.10.1 Clinical Utility

Restricted diffusion on DWI (i.e., high signal intensity on high b-value DWI and low signal intensity on the ADC map) can identify bowel wall inflammation, lymphadenopathy, infected fluid collections, or fibrosis [75]. Also, when bowel inflammation is identified on conventional contrast-enhanced and/or T2-weighted images, the presence of restricted diffusion on DWI may indicate more severe inflammation [8, 9, 46].

4.2.10.2 Advantages

DWI sequences have high contrast resolution which improves identification of pathologic processes when interpreted with other pulse sequences. If gadolinium is contraindicated, DWI becomes especially important in demonstrating bowel inflammation.

4.2.10.3 Disadvantages

Non-breath-hold DWI has a long series acquisition time and can take up to 3–6 min to obtain. Similar to the other series in an MRE exam (except for T2-weighted images), DWI is prone to susceptibility artifact created by metallic structures or bowel gas. Low spatial resolution and limited morphologic information are additional limitations of DWI. Finally, DWI has low specificity for mural inflammation in Crohn's disease, and thus, the findings on DWI should be supplementary to findings on conventional contrast-enhanced and/or T2-weighted images [45, 46, 76].

4.3 CT Enterography

4.3.1 Patient Preparation

Prior to CT enterography (CTE), patients are generally required to fast for 4 h [5, 77, 78]. Fasting helps to ensure that intraluminal ingested material is not confused for intestinal pathology. In order to distend the small bowel and optimize tissue contrast, a neutral oral contrast agent is administered beginning at least 1 h prior to imaging. Neutral oral contrast agents accomplish bowel distention without increasing luminal density (like positive oral contrast agents such as standard barium and iodine solutions). The relative luminal hypodensity increases the conspicuity of the adjacent bowel wall and mural enhancement (Fig. 4.3) [19, 20]. As discussed above, neutral contrast agents include low-density barium sulfate suspension (Volumen), mannitol, sorbitol, polyethylene glycol, water, methylcellulose, and locust bean gum. Because bowel distention is critically important to evaluate bowel wall thickening and enhancement, consuming at least 1 L of contrast agent is recommended. A typical preparation includes administering one bottle of 450 mL of low-density barium sulfate suspension every 20 min beginning 1 h prior to the examination for a total of 1350 mL.

4.3.2 CT Enterography Protocol

In addition to adequate luminal distention, CTE requires intravenous contrast administration and adequate spatial resolution for image postprocessing. For routine studies to evaluate inflammatory bowel disease, a single post-contrast phase obtained approximately 50–65 s following the onset of contrast administration is adequate (Table 4.4) [19]. For evaluation of small bowel bleeding, many centers use a multiphase approach such as a bolus-timed arterial phase, an enteric phase (50 seconds after injection) and possibly a delayed phase (90 seconds after injection) [92–95]. Anatomic coverage spans the top of the liver or hemidiaphragms through the lesser trochanters to ensure complete coverage of the bowel. In order to guarantee adequate image quality and allow for postprocessing, CT detector size should be 1.5 mm or lower, and axial images are reconstructed with a section thickness of between 2.0 and 3.0 mm, generally with a matching interval. Reformatted images in the coronal and sagittal planes with section thickness up to 3.0 mm are often overlapping with a lower interval, typically half the section thickness.

4.3.3 CT Enterography Clinical Utility and Limitations

CTE has largely replaced fluoroscopy as the first-line imaging modality for inflammatory bowel disease. CTE and MRE have comparable diagnostic effectiveness for IBD [18], and the relative benefits of CTE are its lower cost, wider availability, image quality reproducibility, shorter image acquisition time, and greater patient

Table 4.4 CT enterography protocol

Parameter	Single phase
Coverage	Liver dome through lesser trochanter
Scan direction	Top to bottom
IV contrast dose	100 mL
IV contrast rate	3–4 mL/s
Saline flush	Yes
Delay	50 s
Oral contrast	Three bottles of low-density barium sulfate suspension (1350 mL)
Detector size	≤1.5 mm

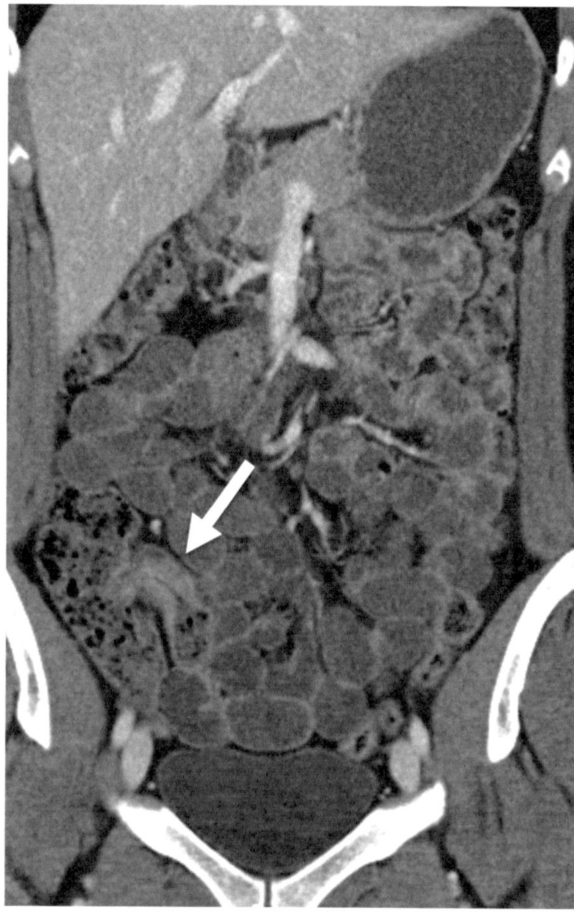

Fig. 4.14 Coronal CT enterography image showing active inflammation with luminal narrowing in the terminal ileum (*arrow*)

acceptance. Because many patients that require a CTE may present earlier in life and require multiple imaging studies, MRE should be the preferred test, except in cases of emergent imaging where the greater ease and availability of CTE is more appropriate and less affected by the patient's clinical condition which may create motion artifact on MRE.

CTE demonstrates findings visible on MRE images in the setting of active inflammation including bowel wall thickening, mural and perienteric edema, segmental mural hyperenhancement, and ulcerations (Fig. 4.14). Associated complications are also readily identifiable including strictures, fistulas and sinus tracts, inflammatory masses, and abscesses (Fig. 4.15).

With image acquisition times of <5 s on modern CT systems, CTE is better adapted to accommodate sick patients without compromising image quality. In addition to coverage advantages, CTE also features high spatial resolution with slice thickness as low as 0.5 mm with matching in-plane resolution, which results in isotropic voxels. This allows for reformatting images with equal image quality in any imaging plane.

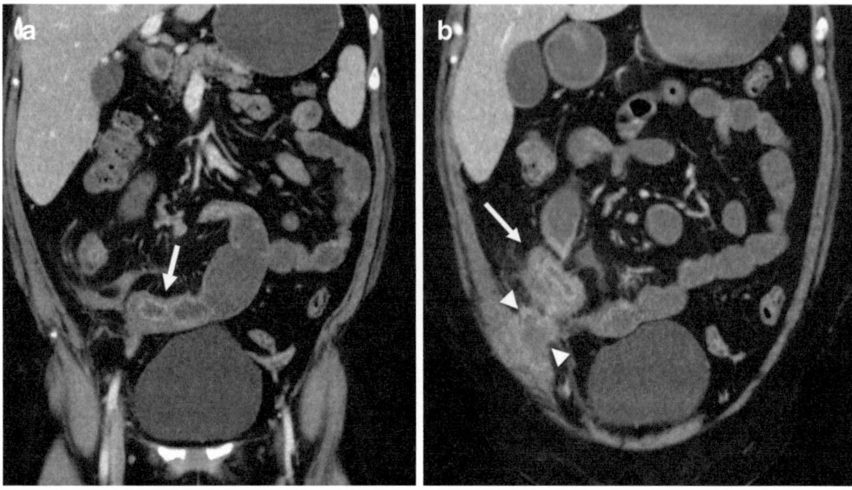

Fig. 4.15 Coronal CT enterography image (**a**) showing wall thickening with increased mural and mucosal enhancement in the terminal ileum (arrows in **a** and **b**) and upstream small bowel dilatation consistent with a stricture with active inflammation. There is an associated adjacent abscess (arrowheads in **b**). There were also fistulas to the adjacent small bowel and appendix (not shown)

One of the main limitations of CTE is the use of ionizing radiation. This is especially important for patients with Crohn's disease due to the recurrent nature of the disease and associated complications which may require multiple imaging studies, potentially resulting in a large cumulative lifetime radiation dose [79–83]. For this reason, radiation dose reduction techniques should routinely be implemented for CTE exams [84]. Methods to reduce CT radiation dose include decreasing the scan coverage, reducing the tube voltage (i.e., kVp), and reducing the tube current product (i.e., mAs). A potential added benefit of reducing the radiation dose by decreasing the tube voltage is more conspicuous hyperenhancement and mural stratification of inflamed bowel segments, thus improving the identification of abnormal bowel segments [84, 85]. The trade-off for reducing the radiation dose by decreasing the tube voltage or tube current product is increased exam noise which can decrease the interpreting radiologist's impression of image quality. However, newer iterative reconstruction techniques and image space denoising techniques can significantly reduce image noise making low-dose images appear similar to higher-dose images regarding image noise levels [29, 85–90]. The combination of low-dose imaging techniques and noise-reduction strategies can result in a substantial decrease in radiation dose while maintaining the diagnostic accuracy of CT exams.

Aside from the radiation dose, the main limitation of CTE compared with MRE is the relatively lower tissue contrast (Fig. 4.1). Tissue contrast in CT is much more dependent on contrast enhancement, and hyperenhancement is less conspicuous with CT than with MRI. Thus, differentiating inflammation and inflammatory masses from abscesses requiring drainage is potentially more difficult (Fig. 4.15).

This limitation significantly limits evaluation of the perianal region and detection of perianal fistulas. Finally, the relatively large quantity of intravenous contrast required to achieve adequate enhancement risks complications such as contrast extravasation or contrast-induced nephropathy in patients that have limited renal function. However, the risk of contrast-induced nephropathy has declined with newer low-osmolar contrast agents compared to the high-osmolar contrast agents used in the past and has likely been inflated by the nature of clinical studies lacking a control group not receiving contrast material [91].

References

1. ACR–SAR–SPR practice parameter for the performance of computed tomography (CT) enterography 2015 (Resolution 18). American College of Radiology. Accessed 15 Jan 2018.
2. Grand DJ, Guglielmo FF, Al-Hawary MM. MR enterography in Crohn's disease: current consensus on optimal imaging technique and future advances from the SAR Crohn's disease-focused panel. Abdom Imaging. 2015;40(5):953–64.
3. ACR–SAR–SPR practice parameter for the performance of magnetic resonance (MR) enterography 2015 (Resolution 9). American College of Radiology. Accessed 15 Jan 2018.
4. Costa-Silva L, Brandão AC. MR enterography for the assessment of small bowel diseases. Magn Reson Imaging Clin N Am. 2013;21(2):365–83.
5. Ilangovan R, Burling D, George A, Gupta A, Marshall M, Taylor S. CT enterography: review of technique and practical tips. Br J Radiol. 2012;85(1015):876–86.
6. Masselli G, Gualdi G. MR imaging of the small bowel. Radiology. 2012;264(2):333–48.
7. Fidler J. MR imaging of the small bowel. Radiol Clin N Am. 2007;45(2):317–31.
8. Bruining DH, Zimmermann EM, Loftus EV Jr, Sandborn WJ, Sauer CG, Strong SA, Society of Abdominal Radiology Crohn's Disease-Focused Panel. Consensus recommendations for evaluation, interpretation, and utilization of computed tomography and magnetic resonance enterography in patients with small bowel Crohn's disease. Radiology. 2018;286(3): 776–99.
9. Bruining DH, Zimmermann EM, Loftus EV, Sandborn WJ, Sauer CG, Strong SA, Society of Abdominal Radiology Crohn's Disease-Focused Panel. Consensus recommendations for evaluation, interpretation, and utilization of computed tomography and magnetic resonance enterography in patients with small bowel Crohn's disease. Gastroenterology. 2018;154(4):1172–94.
10. Amzallag-Bellenger E, Oudjit A, Ruiz A, Cadiot G, Soyer PA, Hoeffel CC. Effectiveness of MR enterography for the assessment of small-bowel diseases beyond Crohn disease. Radiographics. 2012;32(5):1423–44.
11. Fidler JL, Guimaraes L, Einstein DM. MR imaging of the small bowel 1. Radiographics. 2009;29(6):1811–25.
12. Tolan DJ, Greenhalgh R, Zealley IA, Halligan S, Taylor SA. MR enterographic manifestations of small bowel Crohn disease. Radiographics. 2010;30(2):367–84.
13. Laghi A, Paolantonio P, Iafrate F, Altomari F, Miglio C, Passariello R. Oral contrast agents for magnetic resonance imaging of the bowel. Top Magn Reson Imaging. 2002;13(6):389–96.
14. Gee MS, Harisinghani MG. MRI in patients with inflammatory bowel disease. J Magn Reson Imaging. 2011;33(3):527–34.
15. Sinha R, Verma R, Verma S, Rajesh A. MR enterography of Crohn disease: part 1, rationale, technique, and pitfalls. Am J Roentgenol. 2011;197(1):76–9.
16. Griffin N, Grant LA, Anderson S, Irving P, Sanderson J. Small bowel MR enterography: problem solving in Crohn's disease. Insights imaging. 2012;3(3):251–63.
17. Ajaj W, Goehde SC, Schneemann H, Ruehm SG, Debatin JF, Lauenstein TC. Oral contrast agents for small bowel MRI: comparison of different additives to optimize bowel distension. Eur Radiol. 2004;14(3):458–64.

18. Lee SS, Kim AY, Yang S, Chung J, Kim SY, Park SH, et al. Crohn disease of the small bowel: comparison of CT enterography, MR enterography, and small-bowel follow-through as diagnostic techniques. Radiology. 2009;251(3):751–61.
19. Fletcher JG. CT enterography technique: theme and variations. Abdom Imaging. 2009;34(3):283–8.
20. Huprich JE, Fletcher JG. CT enterography: principles, technique and utility in Crohn's disease. Eur J Radiol. 2009;69(3):393–7.
21. Young BM, Fletcher JG, Booya F, Paulsen S, Fidler J, Johnson CD, et al. Head-to-head comparison of oral contrast agents for cross-sectional enterography: small bowel distention, timing, and side effects. J Comput Assist Tomogr. 2008;32(1):32–8.
22. Kolbe AB, Fletcher JG, Froemming AT, Sheedy SP, Koo CW, Pundi K, et al. Evaluation of patient tolerance and small-bowel distention with a new small-bowel distending agent for enterography. Am J Roentgenol. 2016;206(5):994–1002.
23. Rimola J, Rodriguez S, Garcia-Bosch O, Ordas I, Ayala E, Aceituno M, et al. Magnetic resonance for assessment of disease activity and severity in ileocolonic Crohn's disease. Gut. 2009;58(8):1113–20.
24. Koo CW, Shah-Patel LR, Baer JW, Frager DH. Cost-effectiveness and patient tolerance of low-attenuation oral contrast material: milk versus VoLumen. Am J Roentgenol. 2008;190(5):1307–13.
25. Kuehle CA, Ajaj W, Ladd SC, Massing S, Barkhausen J, Lauenstein TC. Hydro-MRI of the small bowel: effect of contrast volume, timing of contrast administration, and data acquisition on bowel distention. Am J Roentgenol. 2006;187(4):W375–85.
26. Siddiki HA, Fidler JL, Fletcher JG, Burton SS, Huprich JE, Hough DM, et al. Prospective comparison of state-of-the-art MR enterography and CT enterography in small-bowel Crohn's disease. Am J Roentgenol. 2009;193(1):113–21.
27. Guglielmo FF, Kania LM, Ahmad HM, Roth CG, Mitchell DG. Interpreting body MRI cases: what you need to know to get started. Abdom Radiol (NY). 2016;41(11):2248–69.
28. Tweedle MF, Kanal E, Muller R. Considerations in the selection of a new gadolinium-based contrast agent. Appl Radiol. 2014;43(5 Suppl):1–11.
29. Baker ME, Hara AK, Platt JF, Maglinte DD, Fletcher JG. CT enterography for Crohn's disease: optimal technique and imaging issues. Abdom Imaging. 2015;40(5):938–52.
30. Schindera ST, Nelson RC, DeLong DM, Jaffe TA, Merkle EM, Paulson EK, et al. Multi–detector row CT of the small bowel: peak enhancement temporal window—initial experience. Radiology. 2007;243(2):438–44.
31. Hussain HK, Londy FJ, Francis IR, Nghiem HV, Weadock WJ, Gebremariam A, et al. Hepatic arterial phase MR imaging with automated bolus-detection three-dimensional fast gradient-recalled-echo sequence: comparison with test-bolus method. Radiology. 2003;226(2):558–66.
32. Mitchell D, Cohen M. MRI Principles. 2nd ed. Philadelphia: Elsevier; 2004.
33. Semelka RC, Helmberger TKG. Contrast agents for MR imaging of the liver. Radiology. 2001;218(1):27–38.
34. Vandenbroucke F, Mortele K, Tatli S, Pelsser V, Erturk S, De Mey J, et al. Noninvasive multidetector computed tomography enterography in patients with small-bowel Crohn's disease: is a 40-second delay better than 70 seconds? Acta Radiol. 2007;48(10):1052–60.
35. Zappa M, Stefanescu C, Cazals-Hatem D, Bretagnol F, Deschamps L, Attar A, et al. Which magnetic resonance imaging findings accurately evaluate inflammation in small bowel Crohn's disease? A retrospective comparison with surgical pathologic analysis. Inflamm Bowel Dis. 2011;17(4):984–93.
36. Makanyanga J, Punwani S, Taylor SA. Assessment of wall inflammation and fibrosis in Crohn's disease: value of T1-weighted gadolinium-enhanced MR imaging. Abdom Imaging. 2012;37(6):933–43.
37. Baker ME, Walter J, Obuchowski NA, Achkar J, Einstein D, Veniero JC, et al. Mural attenuation in normal small bowel and active inflammatory Crohn's disease on CT enterography: location, absolute attenuation, relative attenuation, and the effect of wall thickness. Am J Roentgenol. 2009;192(2):417–23.

38. Grand DJ, Beland M, Harris A. Magnetic resonance enterography. Radiol Clin N Am. 2013;51(1):99–112.
39. Booya F, Fletcher JG, Huprich JE, Barlow JM, Johnson CD, Fidler JL, et al. Active Crohn disease: CT findings and interobserver agreement for enteric phase CT enterography. Radiology. 2006;241(3):787–95.
40. Grand DJ, Kampalath V, Harris A, Patel A, Resnick MB, Machan J, et al. MR enterography correlates highly with colonoscopy and histology for both distal ileal and colonic Crohn's disease in 310 patients. Eur J Radiol. 2012;81(5):e763–9.
41. Grand DJ, Beland MD, Machan JT, Mayo-Smith WW. Detection of Crohn's disease: comparison of CT and MR enterography without anti-peristaltic agents performed on the same day. Eur J Radiol. 2012;81(8):1735–41.
42. Ziech M, Bossuyt P, Laghi A, Lauenstein T, Taylor S, Stoker J. Grading luminal Crohn's disease: which MRI features are considered as important? Eur J Radiol. 2012;81(4):e467–72.
43. Chernish SM, Maglinte DD. Glucagon: common untoward reactions--review and recommendations. Radiology. 1990;177(1):145–6.
44. Gutzeit A, Binkert CA, Koh D, Hergan K, von Weymarn C, Graf N, et al. Evaluation of the anti-peristaltic effect of glucagon and hyoscine on the small bowel: comparison of intravenous and intramuscular drug administration. Eur Radiol. 2012;22(6):1186–94.
45. Park SH. DWI at MR enterography for evaluating bowel inflammation in Crohn disease. Am J Roentgenol. 2016;207(1):40–8.
46. Kim KJ, Lee Y, Park SH, Kang BK, Seo N, Yang SK, et al. Diffusion-weighted MR enterography for evaluating Crohn's disease: how does it add diagnostically to conventional MR enterography? Inflamm Bowel Dis. 2015 Jan;21(1):101–9.
47. Leyendecker JR, Bloomfeld RS, DiSantis DJ, Waters GS, Mott R, Bechtold RE. MR enterography in the management of patients with Crohn disease. Radiographics. 2009;29(6): 1827–46.
48. Cronin CG, Lohan DG, Mhuircheartaigh JN, McKenna D, Alhajeri N, Roche C, et al. MRI small-bowel follow-through: prone versus supine patient positioning for best small-bowel distention and lesion detection. Am J Roentgenol. 2008;191(2):502–6.
49. Guglielmo FF, Mitchell DG, Gupta S. Gadolinium contrast agent selection and optimal use for body MR imaging. Radiol Clin N Am. 2014;52(4):637–56.
50. Santillan CS. MR imaging techniques of the bowel. Magn Reson Imaging Clin N Am. 2014;22(1):1–11.
51. Patak MA, von Weymarn C, Froehlich JM. Small bowel MR imaging: 1.5 T versus 3T. Magn Reson Imaging Clin N Am. 2007;15(3):383–93.
52. Guglielmo FF, Mitchell DG, O'Kane PL, Deshmukh SP, Roth CG, Burach I, et al. Identifying decreased peristalsis of abnormal small bowel segments in Crohn's disease using cine MR enterography: the frozen bowel sign. Abdom Imaging. 2015;40(5):1150–6.
53. Chavhan GB, Babyn PS, Jankharia BG, Cheng HM, Shroff MM. Steady-state MR imaging sequences: physics, classification, and clinical applications. Radiographics. 2008;28(4):1147–60.
54. Scheffler K, Lehnhardt S. Principles and applications of balanced SSFP techniques. Eur Radiol. 2003;13(11):2409–18.
55. Rescinito G, Sirlin C, Cittadini G Jr. Body MRI artefacts: from image degradation to diagnostic utility. Radiol Med. 2009;114(1):18–31.
56. Wnorowski AM, Guglielmo FF, Mitchell DG. How to perform and interpret cine MR enterography. J Magn Reson Imaging. 2015;42(5):1180–9.
57. Froehlich JM, Waldherr C, Stoupis C, Erturk SM, Patak MA. MR motility imaging in Crohn's disease improves lesion detection compared with standard MR imaging. Eur Radiol. 2010;20(8):1945–51.
58. Girometti R, Zuiani C, Toso F, Brondani G, Sorrentino D, Avellini C, et al. MRI scoring system including dynamic motility evaluation in assessing the activity of Crohn's disease of the terminal ileum. Acad Radiol. 2008;15(2):153–64.
59. Menys A, Atkinson D, Odille F, Ahmed A, Novelli M, Rodriguez-Justo M, et al. Quantified terminal ileal motility during MR enterography as a potential biomarker of Crohn's disease activity: a preliminary study. Eur Radiol. 2012;22(11):2494–501.

60. Buhmann-Kirchhoff S, Lang R, Kirchhoff C, Steitz HO, Jauch KW, Reiser M, et al. Functional cine MR imaging for the detection and mapping of intraabdominal adhesions: method and surgical correlation. Eur Radiol. 2008;18(6):1215–23.
61. Lang RA, Buhmann S, Hopman A, Steitz H, Lienemann A, Reiser MF, et al. Cine-MRI detection of intraabdominal adhesions: correlation with intraoperative findings in 89 consecutive cases. Surg Endosc. 2008;22(11):2455–61.
62. Ito K, Mitchell DG, Outwater EK, Szklaruk J, Sadek AG. Hepatic lesions: discrimination of nonsolid, benign lesions from solid, malignant lesions with heavily T2-weighted fast spin-echo MR imaging. Radiology. 1997;204(3):729–37.
63. Guglielmo FF, Mitchell DG, Roth CG, Deshmukh S. Hepatic MR imaging techniques, optimization, and artifacts. Magn Reson Imaging Clin N Am. 2014;22(3):263–82.
64. Udayasankar UK, Martin D, Lauenstein T, Rutherford R, Galloway J, Tudorascu D, et al. Role of spectral presaturation attenuated inversion-recovery fat-suppressed T2-weighted MR imaging in active inflammatory bowel disease. J Magn Reson Imaging. 2008;28(5):1133–40.
65. Merkle EM, Nelson RC. Dual gradient-echo in-phase and opposed-phase hepatic MR imaging: a useful tool for evaluating more than fatty infiltration or fatty sparing. Radiographics. 2006;26(5):1409–18.
66. Earls JP, Krinsky GA. Abdominal and pelvic applications of opposed-phase MR imaging. AJR Am J Roentgenol. 1997 Oct;169(4):1071–7.
67. Ma J. Breath-hold water and fat imaging using a dual-echo two-point Dixon technique with an efficient and robust phase-correction algorithm. Magn Reson Med. 2004;52(2):415–9.
68. Rosenkrantz AB, Mannelli L, Kim S, Babb JS. Gadolinium-enhanced liver magnetic resonance imaging using a 2-point Dixon fat-water separation technique: impact upon image quality and lesion detection. J Comput Assist Tomogr. 2011;35(1):96–101.
69. Koh D, Miao Y, Chinn R, Amin Z, Zeegen R, Westaby D, et al. MR imaging evaluation of the activity of Crohn's disease. Am J Roentgenol. 2001;177(6):1325–32.
70. Sinha R, Rajiah P, Ramachandran I, Sanders S, Murphy PD. Diffusion-weighted MR imaging of the gastrointestinal tract: technique, indications, and imaging findings. Radiographics. 2013;33(3):655–76.
71. Seo N, Park SH, Kim K, Kang B, Lee Y, Yang S, et al. MR enterography for the evaluation of small-bowel inflammation in Crohn disease by using diffusion-weighted imaging without intravenous contrast material: a prospective noninferiority study. Radiology. 2015;278(3):762–72.
72. Oto A, Kayhan A, Williams JT, Fan X, Yun L, Arkani S, et al. Active Crohn's disease in the small bowel: evaluation by diffusion weighted imaging and quantitative dynamic contrast enhanced MR imaging. J Magn Reson Imaging. 2011;33(3):615–24.
73. Oto A, Zhu F, Kulkarni K, Karczmar GS, Turner JR, Rubin D. Evaluation of diffusion-weighted MR imaging for detection of bowel inflammation in patients with Crohn's disease. Acad Radiol. 2009;16(5):597–603.
74. Kiryu S, Dodanuki K, Takao H, Watanabe M, Inoue Y, Takazoe M, et al. Free-breathing diffusion-weighted imaging for the assessment of inflammatory activity in Crohn's disease. J Magn Reson Imaging. 2009;29(4):880–6.
75. Tielbeek JA, Ziech ML, Li Z, Lavini C, Bipat S, Bemelman WA, et al. Evaluation of conventional, dynamic contrast enhanced and diffusion weighted MRI for quantitative Crohn's disease assessment with histopathology of surgical specimens. Eur Radiol. 2014;24(3):619–29.
76. Rimola J, Alvarez-Cofiño A, Pérez-Jeldres T, Rodríguez S, Alfaro I, Ordás I, et al. Increasing efficiency of MRE for diagnosis of Crohn's disease activity through proper sequence selection: a practical approach for clinical trials. Abdom Radiol (NY). 2017;42(12):2783–91.
77. CT Enterography. RadiologyInfo.org. Accessed 25 Nov 2017.
78. Paulsen SR, Huprich JE, Fletcher JG, Booya F, Young BM, Fidler JL, et al. CT enterography as a diagnostic tool in evaluating small bowel disorders: review of clinical experience with over 700 cases. Radiographics. 2006;26(3):641–57.
79. Chatu S, Subramanian V, Pollok R. Meta-analysis: diagnostic medical radiation exposure in inflammatory bowel disease. Aliment Pharmacol Ther. 2012;35(5):529–39.

80. Desmond AN, O'Regan K, Curran C, McWilliams S, Fitzgerald T, Maher MM, et al. Crohn's disease: factors associated with exposure to high levels of diagnostic radiation. Gut. 2008;57(11):1524–9.
81. Jaffe TA, Gaca AM, Delaney S, Yoshizumi TT, Toncheva G, Nguyen G, et al. Radiation doses from small-bowel follow-through and abdominopelvic MDCT in Crohn's disease. Am J Roentgenol. 2007;189(5):1015–22.
82. Kroeker KI, Lam S, Birchall I, Fedorak RN. Patients with IBD are exposed to high levels of ionizing radiation through CT scan diagnostic imaging: a five-year study. J Clin Gastroenterol. 2011;45(1):34–9.
83. Peloquin JM, Pardi DS, Sandborn WJ, Fletcher JG, McCollough CH, Schueler BA, et al. Diagnostic ionizing radiation exposure in a population-based cohort of patients with inflammatory bowel disease. Am J Gastroenterol. 2008;103(8):2015–22.
84. Mayo-Smith WW, Hara AK, Mahesh M, Sahani DV, Pavlicek W. How I do it: managing radiation dose in CT. Radiology. 2014;273(3):657–72.
85. Del Gaizo AJ, Fletcher JG, Yu L, Paden RG, Spencer GC, Leng S, et al. Reducing radiation dose in CT enterography. Radiographics. 2013;33(4):1109–24.
86. Allen BC, Baker ME, Einstein DM, Remer EM, Herts BR, Achkar J, et al. Effect of altering automatic exposure control settings and quality reference mAs on radiation dose, image quality, and diagnostic efficacy in MDCT enterography of active inflammatory Crohn's disease. Am J Roentgenol. 2010;195(1):89–100.
87. Guimarães LS, Fletcher JG, Yu L, Huprich JE, Fidler JL, Manduca A, et al. Feasibility of dose reduction using novel denoising techniques for low kV (80 kV) CT enterography: optimization and validation. Acad Radiol. 2010;17(10):1203–10.
88. Hough DM, Fletcher JG, Grant KL, Fidler JL, Yu L, Geske JR, et al. Lowering kilovoltage to reduce radiation dose in contrast-enhanced abdominal CT: initial assessment of a prototype automated kilovoltage selection tool. Am J Roentgenol. 2012;199(5):1070–7.
89. Kaza RK, Platt JF, Al-Hawary MM, Wasnik A, Liu PS, Pandya A. CT enterography at 80 kVp with adaptive statistical iterative reconstruction versus at 120 kVp with standard reconstruction: image quality, diagnostic adequacy, and dose reduction. Am J Roentgenol. 2012;198(5):1084–92.
90. Gonzalez-Guindalini FD, Botelho MPF, Töre HG, Ahn RW, Gordon LI, Yaghmai V. MDCT of chest, abdomen, and pelvis using attenuation-based automated tube voltage selection in combination with iterative reconstruction: an intrapatient study of radiation dose and image quality. Am J Roentgenol. 2013;201(5):1075–82.
91. Davenport MS, Cohan RH, Khalatbari S, Ellis JH. The challenges in assessing contrast-induced nephropathy: where are we now? Am J Roentgenol. 2014;202(4):784–9.
92. James E. Huprich, John M. Barlow, Stephanie L. Hansel, Jeffrey A. Alexander, Jeff L. Fidler. Multiphase CT enterography evaluation of small-bowel vascular lesions. Am J Roentgenol. 2013;201(1):65–72.
93. Soto JA, Park SH, Fletcher JG, Fidler JL. Gastrointestinal hemorrhage: evaluation with MDCT. Abdom Imaging. 2015;40(5):993–1009.
94. Wells ML, Hansel SL, Bruining DH, Fletcher JG, Froemming AT, Barlow JM, et al. CT for evaluation of acute gastrointestinal bleeding. Radiographics. 2018;38(4):1089–107.
95. Kim G, Soto JA, Morrison T. Radiologic assessment of gastrointestinal bleeding. Gastroenterol Clin North Am. 2018;47(3):501–14.

MR Enterography and CT Enterography for Detecting Activity and Complications

5

Ragna Vanslembrouck

5.1 Introduction

Crohn's disease (CD) is one of the major subtypes of inflammatory bowel disease (IBD) and can occur in the whole digestive tract, from the mouth to the anus, most commonly in the ileocolonic region. Periods of active inflammation with clinical symptoms alternating with periods of clinical remission are typical for this disease. IBD is caused by an immune dysregulation of the digestive tract and results in chronic inflammation. Persistent mucosal inflammation is thought to be the basis of progressive and disabling bowel damage. Typical symptoms of abdominal pain, cramping, diarrhea, bloody stools, weight loss, fever, and fatigue can result in a decreased quality of life. The severity and chronicity of this disease can lead to severe bowel wall destruction with the development of strictures and internal penetrating disease, a potential source of great morbidity.

Assessment of disease location, extension, activity, and severity of inflammation is important for clinical management. Several studies demonstrated a poor correlation between clinical symptoms, endoscopic findings, and biological activity in CD. It is well established that the CD activity index (CDAI) and the C-reactive protein (CRP) do not reflect the intestinal lesions in CD. A new "treat-to-target" strategy is based on the hypothesis that the treatment of endoscopic mucosal inflammation not only improves symptoms but also decreases the long-term burden of disease. It is important to detect active inflammatory lesions and determine the severity, because data have reported that mucosal healing is correlated with better disease prognosis: less disease relapses, less hospitalizations, and less surgery [1–3].

Currently, endoscopy is the most essential study, the golden standard, in the diagnosis and assessment of IBD but has several limitations, such as the invasiveness, the risk of complications, the difficulty to perform total ileocolonoscopy in case of

R. Vanslembrouck (✉)
Department of Radiology, University Hospitals Leuven, Leuven, Belgium
e-mail: ragna.vanslembrouck@uzleuven.be

J. Rimola (ed.), *Cross-Sectional Imaging in Crohn's Disease*,
https://doi.org/10.1007/978-3-319-96586-4_5

stenosis and adhesions or severity of inflammatory lesions (the right colon can be explored in 90% of subjects, and it decreases to 75% for the terminal ileum) [4], and the impossibility to visualize the whole bowel wall and extraintestinal complications.

The small bowel follow-through and enteroclysis used to be the radiological imaging methods of choice for evaluating the small bowel in CD, but since the increasing development of cross-sectional imaging techniques in the last decades, CTE and MRE have become vital tools and the most effective methods in the non-invasive assessment of small bowel in patients with CD, complementary to endoscopy and biopsy.

5.2 Imaging Findings of CD Activity and Complications into Imaging Findings of CD Activity and Complications on CT Enterography and MR Enterography

5.2.1 Active Inflammation

Several parameters suggest active inflammation in Crohn's disease (CD) on both CTE and MRE, including increased mucosal hyperenhancement, bowel wall thickening, ulcerations, mural hyperenhancement, and mural stratification [5–8].

Increased mucosal enhancement/hyperenhancement (Fig. 5.2b, c) is one of the earliest signs of activity on MRE and is associated with mild to moderate edema. It can be seen with or without bowel wall thickening.

In the early stage of active inflammation discrete mucosal lesions, such as aphtoïd lesions, erythema, friability, and other non-ulcerative lesions are present. Even in a well-distended bowel loop, aphtoïd lesions are not visible on both CTE and MRE, neither on CT enteroclysis nor MR enteroclysis where more bowel distention is obtained.

In the progression of active disease, deep ulcers develop and penetrate into the deep layers of the bowel wall, the submucosa, resulting in submucosal infiltration of inflammatory cells and edema. The presence of ulcerations suggests severe inflammation. Longitudinal and transverse ulcerations surrounding inflamed but not ulcerated mucosa create "cobblestoning" or inflammatory pseudopolyps (Fig. 5.1c). The latter are easily seen in a well-distended bowel on CTE and MRE as contrast-enhancing nodules. The presence of "cobblestoning" is suggestive of advanced and severe CD.

In an optimal distended bowel loop, mural thickening is present when the bowel wall is greater than 3 mm. Mural thickening (Fig. 5.1a, b) is an important finding of active CD inflammation. It can be caused by inflammatory cell infiltration, bowel wall edema, and/or fibrosis. Bowel wall edema can be detected on MRE as a high signal in the submucosa on T2-weighted images (T2-WI) and is suggestive of severe inflammation, although the absence of this increased T2 signal does not exclude the presence of active inflammation. Submucosal high signal on the T2-WI can be caused by edema or by infiltration of fat (Fig. 5.2a–c), which can be differentiated by performing additional T2 fat suppression sequences. The high signal on T2 will remain high on the fat-saturated images in case of edema, and there will be a signal drop, if submucosal fat deposition is present, suggestive of chronic inflammation.

The degree of bowel wall thickening is correlated with the severity of CD inflammation.

Increased bowel wall attenuation (Fig. 5.1a, b), compared to adjacent normal small bowel loops, is nonspecific but one of the most sensitive CT and MR findings for active CD inflammation. These parameters can be asymmetrical, due to the preferential inflammatory involvement of the mesenteric side of the bowel wall (Fig. 5.4a), and the latter is probably a characteristic finding in CD [9].

Mural stratification (Fig. 5.1a, b) is a three-layered pattern of contrast enhancement and consists of strong enhancement of the mucosa, relatively poor-enhancing submucosa and strong enhancement of the serosa [10].

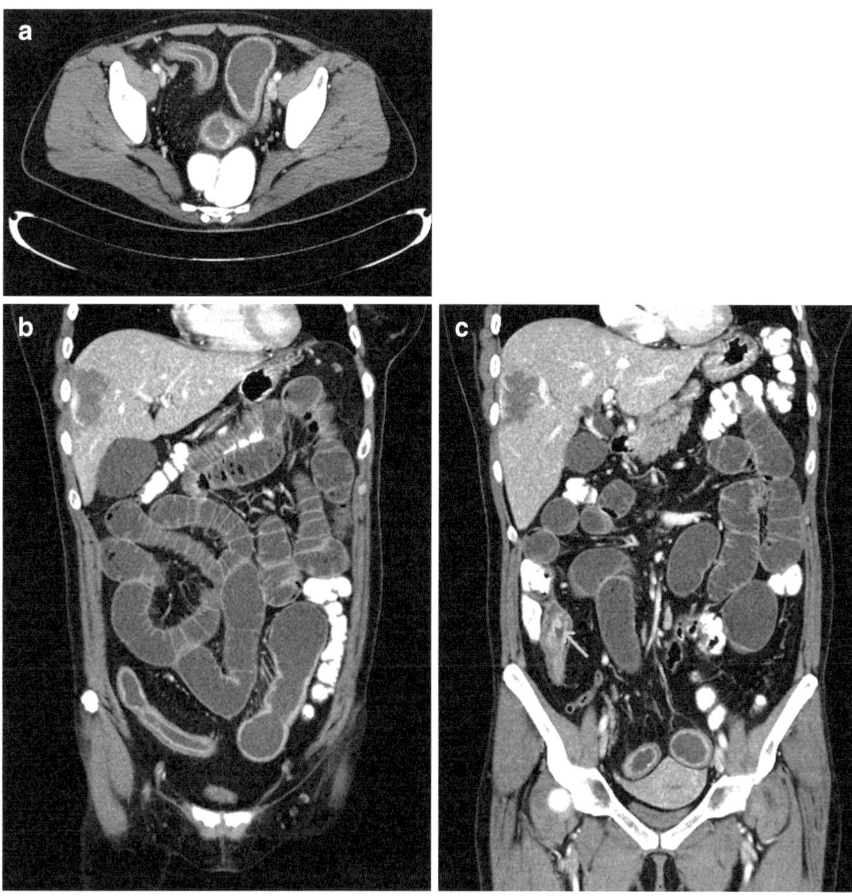

Fig. 5.1 A 53-year-old female patient with severe, extensive, active Crohn's disease in the ileum on CT enterography with the following mural and extramural features: circumferential wall thickening, increased mural enhancement, mucosal hyperenhancement, mural stratification, enhancing pseudopolyp (arrow on the coronal image, **c**), "comb sign," and fibrofatty proliferation

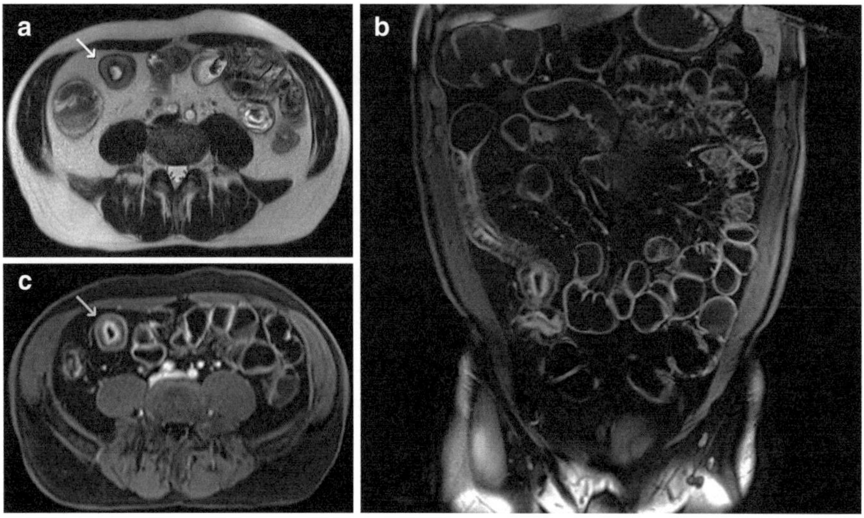

Fig. 5.2 A 55-year-old man with severe, extensive, stenotic, and long-standing active-on-chronic CD in the ileum and right colectomy. Axial T2 HASTE image (**a**) shows an important wall thickening of the ileum with important submucosal fat infiltration (*arrow*), suggesting long-standing CD. Coronal (**b**) and axial (**c**) fat-suppressed 3D T1 GRE images show a stenotic distal ileal segment with severe wall thickening, mucosal hyperenhancement, mural stratification (*arrow*), "comb sign," and fibrofatty proliferation

Associated CT and MR parameters suggesting active inflammation include increased mesenteric fat density and increased T2 intensity due to inflammation of the mesenteric fat or mesenteric edema surrounding the inflamed bowel segments and free fluid. Edema in the mesenteric fat and the presence of free fluid on MRE is best detected on the T2-WI with fat suppression, as a permanent high T2 signal.

Dilated vasa recta, so-called comb sign, is created by the perpendicular passage of engorged vasa recta vessels to the bowel lumen and is the result of increased blood flow through the vasa recta to the inflamed bowel segments (Fig. 5.4a). The "comb sign" has been reported to be associated with higher C-reactive protein levels and more intensive medical therapy compared to CD patients with normal vasculature [11].

Increased attenuation of the mesenteric fat and "comb sign" both correlate with clinically advanced, active, and extensive CD.

Fibrofatty proliferation is another characteristic feature, appearing as an increased quantity of mesenteric fat, producing a mass effect on adjacent loops, predominantly along the mesenteric side of the bowel, as a result of edema and infiltration of inflammatory cells in the perienteric fat. Fibrofatty proliferation may persist in non-active CD.

Enlarged and increased enhancing mesenteric lymph nodes are frequently seen in patients with active and inactive CD, often surrounding the diseased bowel segments, especially around the ileocolic vessels, given the preferred side of CD inflammation (Fig. 5.3b).

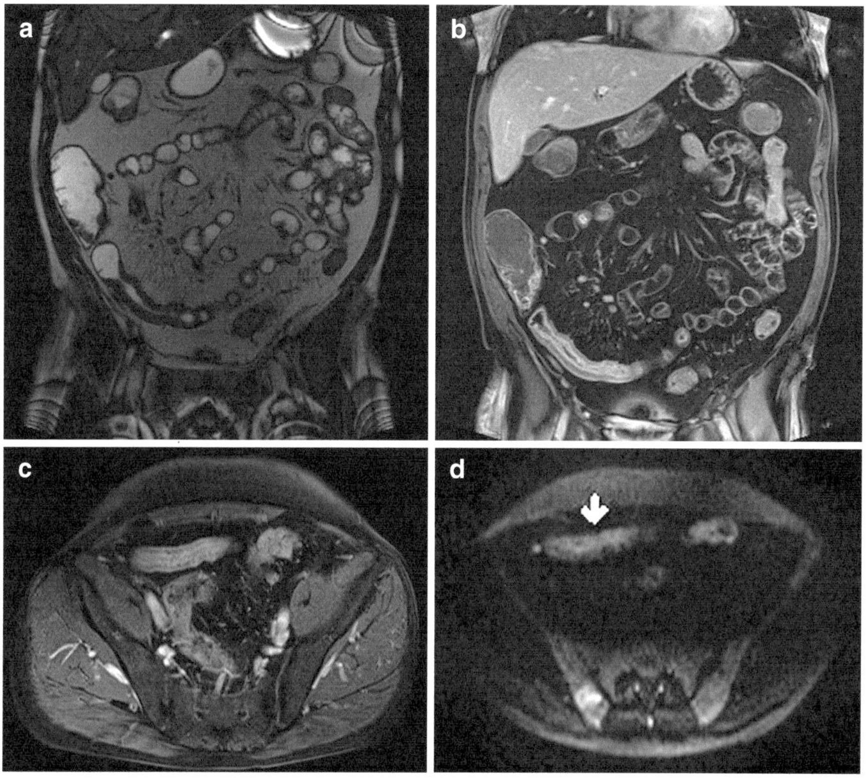

Fig. 5.3 A 55-year-old man with active CD inflammation of the distal ileum. Coronal true FISP image (**a**) shows severe wall thickening, "comb sign," and lymph nodes in the adjacent mesenteric fat. Coronal (**b**) and axial (**c**) fat-suppressed 3D T1 GRE images show additional increased mural enhancement, mucosal hyperenhancement, and mural stratification. Axial diffusion-weighted image (**d**) with *b*-value of 1200 s/mm^2, consistent with restricted diffusion (*arrow*). Overall findings are indicative of active inflammation

In our experience the presence of "comb sign" and/or increased number of lymph nodes can help in the detection of bowel inflammation in under-dilated bowel segments, often the case in jejunal and/or proximal ileal bowel loops, where wall thickness is not so evident compared to distal small bowel segments.

A prospective study with 100 patients with mild and moderate disease evaluated small intestinal CD lesions by comparing MR enterocolonography (MREC) with enteroscopic findings in the jejunum and proximal ileum [12]. This study showed good diagnostic accuracy for the detection of lesions of any degree of severity in the small intestine. There was no significant difference in the sensitivity and specificity for active lesions in the terminal ileum compared to the other small intestinal segments. They suggest the need for assessing CD lesions in deep small intestine, given their comparable endoscopic detection of active lesions, not only in the terminal ileum but also in the more proximal ileal segments, and their mild correlation between (active) endoscopic lesions and the CDAI. Another study from the same group also found a positive correlation between endoscopic and MaRIA scores for the detection of lesions of any degree of severity in the small intestine [13]. MRE has proven to be useful for detecting active disease and assessing the severity of CD lesions, but most of the data has been derived from comparing endoscopic findings from the terminal ileum and colon.

A recent retrospective study compared imaging features on CTE and MRE in histologically proven active CD in children and adolescents [14]. Two mural imaging features, thickening of the bowel wall and hyperenhancement, were evaluated, both performed similarly well on CTE and MRE. On the other hand, the perienteric features evaluated in this study, comb sign, perienteric edema, and fibrofatty proliferation, performed worse on MRE compared to CTE. These results suggest that the mural abnormalities are more reliable imaging findings on both CTE and MRE, whereas perienteric features, which rely on the visualization of smaller structures, are less reliable on MRE compared to CTE. The latter can be explained by the fact that there are a decrease in spatial resolution, a higher susceptibility to motion artifacts, and a higher variability in image quality on MRE compared to CTE.

Diffusion-weighted imaging (DWI) can differentiate an inflamed bowel from a normal bowel. On DWI, an inflamed bowel wall is restricted i.e. appearing brighter on these T2-weighted images compared to a normal bowel (Fig. 5.3c, d). Diffusion restriction is a nonspecific sign of CD bowel wall inflammation, but when other typical findings of CD bowel wall inflammation are present on T2-WI and/or on the contrast-enhanced T1-weighted images (T1-WI), then restricted diffusion is an additional finding that is suggestive for severe CD inflammation.

Apparent diffusion coefficient (ADC) mapping permits quantitative assessment of these sequences. It is still not clear if DWI has an added value over the standard T2-WI and the dynamic contrast-enhanced imaging.

Multiple studies have evaluated the accuracy of DWI in the diagnosis and determination of the severity of active inflammation in CD [15, 16]. Most studies suggest a high degree of accuracy in CD evaluation. It has been suggested that DWI, alone or in combination with other sequences, especially T2-WI and intravenous contrast-enhanced T1-WI, can increase MRE's sensitivity in detecting active inflammation, especially for lesions with mild severity [17–19].

The accuracy of DWI is more variable and lower in the colon than in the small bowel, mainly the specificity; this may be explained by the presence of air in the colon lumen, creating more artifacts. The latter may be reduced by better colon preparation and a water enema.

DWI can in some cases be used as an alternative to gadolinium [15, 18], such as in patients allergic to gadolinium, decreased renal function, and pregnancy. However, well-distended and well-prepared bowel areas are needed to avoid DWI-MRE false-positive results. DWI is a sequence with relatively long acquisition time (making it more sensitive to bowel motion) which may be reduced with intravenous antiperistaltic agents before imaging. Another disadvantage is the presence of T2 shine-through effects, spontaneous high signal intensity of bowel content, present in the bowel lumen [16]. ADC can differentiate between diffusion restriction and T2 shine-through: ADC will be low in case of diffusion restriction and high in case of

T2 shine-through. The latter can be reduced by using high *b*-values and short echo times. The use of respiratory triggering or free-breathing acquisition is variable.

5.2.2 Stricturing Disease

A stricture is a small bowel segment with narrowing of the bowel lumen and prestenotic dilated bowel. Upstream dilation is a helpful tool in suggesting a fixed or a transient stricture.

In patients with active CD, stenotic bowel lesions or strictures may occur due to bowel wall infiltration of inflammatory cells, edema, and bowel spasm but are more frequently present in patients with fibrostenosing disease due to fibrosis and muscle hypertrophy [6–8, 11]. Dynamic contrast-enhanced sequences on MRE provide additional information compared to CTE, especially in terms of any possibility to differentiate active inflamed bowel wall from fibrotic tissue. Active inflammatory strictures are represented with mural hyperenhancement, more severe bowel wall thickening, and mural stratification, whereas chronic fibrostenotic strictures are represented with a thinner wall, hypointense on T1 and T2 sequences, absence of edema and local "comb sign," lower bowel wall enhancement, and possible submucosal fat deposition, a sign of chronic disease [20]. An increased retention of contrast in fibrotic tissue is seen on the delayed phase sequences.

Differentiating active from chronic strictures is important for therapeutic management. Active strictures are generally treated medically and chronic strictures in most of the patients surgically or by endoscopy depending on the length, location, and aspect of the stenotic lesion. Short stenosis with a non-curved shape, within the reach for endoscopy, can easily be dilated. However active disease and fibrosis are often found in the same patient and even in the same diseased bowel segments, so superimposed mucosal enhancement may be present in fibrotic strictures. The majority of strictures in CD have both an inflammatory and fibrotic portion secondary to repeated inflammation and repair [9]. A recent, prospective, unicentric study of 31 patients showed good results in differentiating fibrotic from inflammatory strictures and in distinguishing different grades of fibrosis, by using magnetization transfer imaging, compared to contrast-enhanced MRE sequences and DWI, with histopathologic evaluation as reference standard [21].

It remains difficult to estimate what is most present in which stricture, in terms of the contribution of inflammation, fibrosis, and smooth muscle hypertrophy. A lot of research has been done on this topic, but none of the investigated imaging techniques has been completely validated.

DWI is restricted in both inflammatory and fibrotic strictures, and ADC measurements don't seem to help to differentiate them [16].

A benefit of MRE over CTE is that multiphase cine imaging allows assessment of bowel motility and can offer additional information in the differentiation between fixed stenotic lesions and temporary luminal narrowing. Bowel dilatation proximal to a stenotic segment helps confirm the functional importance of this stenotic segment, although not all bowel dilatation is related to fibrotic strictures. When a fixed stricture with obstruction is present distal to a fistula, the fistula is not going to close as long as the fixed stricture occurs [20].

In addition, strictures should be evaluated carefully to exclude or identify underlying malignant tumor, considering the increased incidence of bowel malignancies in patients with CD [9].

All previous features are important and they influence therapeutic decision-making.

Penetrating and stricturing disease are strongly associated. Penetrating disease occurs strongly in patients with strictures associated with active inflammation. When a fistula is detected, an inflamed and stenotic bowel segment with prestenotic dilatation is nearly always present. Penetrating complications are nearly always present at the proximal side of the stricture.

5.2.3 Penetrating Disease

As disease progresses, deep ulcers penetrate through the whole bowel wall, extending in the adjacent mesenteric fat and creating a sinus tract. A sinus tract ends blind, becoming a fistula tract when connecting with other bowel loops or structures (Fig. 5.4b). A fistula can be single or complex with multiple tracts, with angulated or tethered aspect of the affected bowel loops (Fig. 5.5a, b). These fistulas can further complicate in an inflammatory mass or an abscess and rarely in a free intraperitoneal perforation. The presence of sinus tracts and fistulas indicates severe active CD.

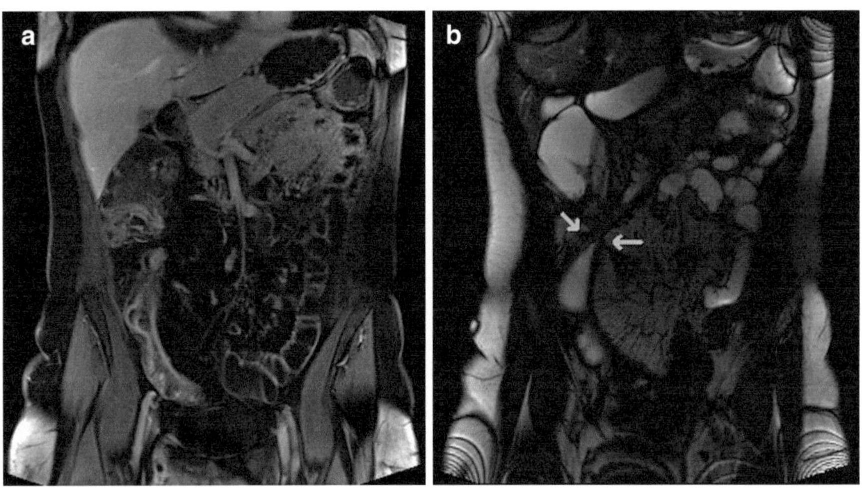

Fig. 5.4 A 36-year-old female patient with severe, extensive, long-standing active-on-chronic CD in the distal ileum. Coronal fat-suppressed 3D T1 GRE image (**a**) with pseudosacculation of the antimesenteric wall of the inflamed ileal segment. Coronal true FISP image (**b**) shows complex fistulas between ileal loops, with angulated and tethered aspect or "star sign"

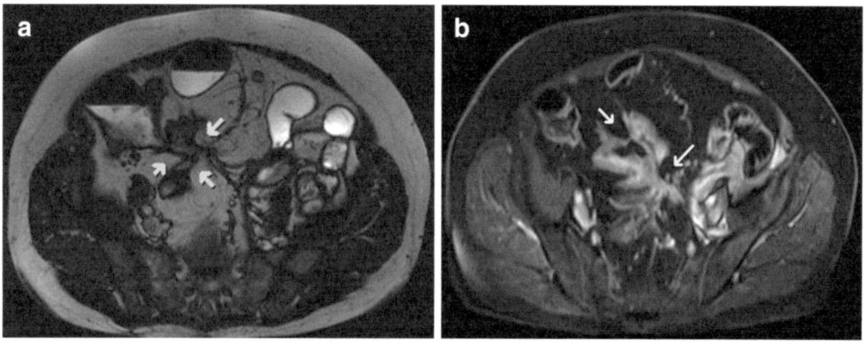

Fig. 5.5 A 52-year-old female patient with severe, long-standing active-on-chronic ileal CD. Axial true FISP image (**a**) and axial fat-suppressed 3D T1 GRE image (**b**) show complex fistulas between ileal and sigmoid loops in the adjacent mesenteric fat, with tethered aspect or "star sign"

A sinus tract is a blind-ending inflammatory tract that can connect with another structure, fluid-filled cavity, intra- or extra-abdominal space, becoming a fistula. On CTE and MRE, they present as linear or tubular contrast-enhancing tracts without or with connection to, for example, other bowel segments (small bowel, colon, and stomach), bladder, abdominal wall, skin, retroperitoneum and others [6–8]. Fistulas are well seen with DWI.

The perianal fistula is the most common fistula in CD (see Chap. 8).

Recent data report a higher incidence of perienteric mesenteric inflammation and perienteric fluid collection in patients with enteroenteric fistula, caused by rupture of lymphatic vessels or reactive to the inflammation in the surrounding tissues [22]. Enteroenteric fistula should not be confused with peritoneal adhesions, which are often seen in CD and can cause bowel obstruction. Fistula is thicker and enhances faster than fibrotic adhesions [6]. When enteroenteric fistula heals, a fibrotic adhesion to the bowels may replace the fistula tract. It is mentioned that there is a difference in the amount and aspect of the mesenteric fat surrounding adhesive and fistulizing bowel loops: more mesenteric fat is seen between adhesive bowel loops, and less fat with more beak-like appearance is more frequently seen in fistulizing bowel segments [22].

An abscess is mostly present in the mesenterium, adjacent to the inflamed bowel, but can, for example, also develop in the retroperitoneal space or in the abdominal wall. Abscesses can easily be detected on both CTE and MRE, but CT is often the first-line examination in acute settings due to limited MRI access and longer examination time compared to CT. An abscess is well detected on DWI, the pus restricts the diffusion of water, and ADC values are low.

The detection of the presence of an abscess is crucial and can change treatment management.

Other extraintestinal findings related to CD can be visualized on CTE and MRE, such as venous thrombosis of mesenteric veins, portal veins, primary sclerosing cholangitis, cholecystolithiasis, sacroiliitis, and avascular necrosis, mostly of the femoral heads [9].

MRE is mostly performed for the evaluation of small bowel CD; the colon can be evaluated with endoscopy, with the exception of the presence of a stenotic lesion in the colon that can't be passed by the scope. Features of active and chronic inflammation are comparable with those seen in the small bowel.

5.3 Diagnostic Accuracy

The optimal imaging technique should be able to detect and grade activity with high accuracy and also has the possibility to detect enteric and extraenteric complications.

CT is a quick accessible, reliable, and fast technique, with better spatial resolution than MR, and is seen as the most appropriate imaging technique for the evaluation of patients with CD.

Despite several efforts to lower the radiation dose, the use of ionizing radiation and the need for repetitive imaging during the course of CD are great concerns, especially because the population consists of young patients. The radiation exposure has been considered the main drawback of CT imaging.

So MRE is in certain settings the first-line radiation-free imaging technique for the evaluation of CD. MR provides better soft tissue contrast. MRE allows the assessment of the complete digestive tract and offers great patient acceptance and good reproducibility. The limitations of MRI are the relatively high cost, the overall lack of availability, low spatial resolution, and susceptibility to artifacts, although these technical limitations have been reduced to a minimum in recent years. Differences in types of imaging equipment and MRE scanning protocols have to be considered, such as bowel filling, image quality, and the use of additional sequences, such as DWI, cine MRE, etc. Another consideration is the availability of the necessary expertise of the radiologist to perform and interpret CTE and MRE images.

Accurate evaluation of the small bowel on CTE and MRE requires good bowel distention, obtained with oral contrast. Better bowel distention can be achieved with CT and MR enteroclysis, but a few technical disadvantages, such as the need for radiation exposure during the placement of the nasojejunal tube and patients' discomfort, made us, in our institution, nearly abandon this technique. We rarely perform MR enteroclysis in cases of suspected proximal small bowel CD inaccessible with endoscopy or if insufficient bowel distension can be achieved with oral contrast.

Multiple studies revealed that CT and MRI both have a high diagnostic accuracy in the detection of active small bowel CD and that there is no statistically significant difference between CT and MR in the detection and assessment of small bowel CD activity and complications [23, 24]. There is also a high accuracy for detecting postoperative recurrence for both techniques, especially when there is a stenotic anastomosis, impossible to evaluate adequate with endoscopy.

Individual signs of active inflammation have varying sensitivity and specificity and they are all useful. CTE is highly accurate in detecting bowel wall thickening, evaluating bowel wall enhancement, and detecting aforementioned local vascular and mesenteric changes. MRE is very accurate in detecting mural thickening, mucosal and mural hyperenhancement, mural edema, "comb sign," mesenteric changes, and lymph nodes. Compared to a surgical resection specimen, there is a good correlation with the presence of strictures, fistulas, and abscesses, compared to findings both on CTE and MRE. A limitation in detecting early mucosal disease, both on CTE and MRE, even with good bowel distention, was mentioned in several studies. In studies evaluating the detection of intramural fibrosis, there is definitely a role for MRE, but reliable data is still missing.

Bowel wall enhancement and bowel wall thickening are most specific for active inflammation. DWI is very sensitive for detecting activity; data have suggested that the combination of T2 sequences and DWI can accurately detect activity without the need for gadolinium [19]. Although DWI is very sensitive in detecting activity, it reduces the specificity of MRE [15, 18, 19]. DWI is inadequate as a stand-alone technique but can be helpful when combined with other sequences: it may increase MRE sensitivity for detecting inflammation, especially for non-severe lesions [17–19]. Wall thickening (>3 mm), edema, and ulcerations are very specific for severe CD, and edema is most specific [19]. Perienteric inflammation is probably also specific for severity. The more individual signs are present and the more the most relevant are present, the more severe the disease. Other signs like lymph nodes, "comb sign," and motility are not so specific because these features also depend on location, duration of the disease, age of patient, and other factors.

Detecting activity is not sufficient to guide therapeutic decision making; disease severity is a crucial factor in most of the current therapeutic algorithms.

The presence or absence of ulcerative lesions is an important factor as end point of the disease given their prognosis in the course of the disease, hospitalizations, and the need for surgery.

In a prospective study of 50 patients with mild and severe active and inactive ileocolonic CD, Rimola et al. compared several MR parameters of active inflammation with endoscopic findings, to determine the MR signs that best describe the presence of endoscopically active disease and the presence of severe disease, and proposed the magnetic resonance index of activity (MaRIA) that highly correlated with endoscopic disease [25]. These MR parameters are wall thickness, relative contrast enhancement, and the presence of edema and ulcerations. There is a cutoff value of 7 or more for determining active disease and a cutoff value of 11 or more for the assessment of presence of severe disease, in a segment-by-segment analysis. The evaluation of wall thickness and the assessment of relative contrast enhancement (RCE) are essential for the detection of active inflammation, but the presence of edema and ulcerations is necessary for the assessment of the severity of the inflammation. This index underwent an internal and external validation in an independent cohort [26]. Although this score does not reflect the overall burden of disease, it can be considered as the most validated tool for assessing CD inflammation by MR. This and other proposed scoring systems, such as Clermont score and MEGS, are used in clinical studies to give a quantitative indication of active inflammatory CD's improvement or the opposite. A more simplified version of these scores is preferable for the use in daily practice.

5.4 Assessment of Treatment Response

The therapy end points for CD are developing gradually over the years [27, 28] because of the growing availability of therapeutic options for the treatment of IBD.

The goal of treatment would be trying to change the natural history of IBD by preventing and delaying disease progression.

Remission in IBD is still evolving. The state of remission could be defined as a state without biological evidence of inflammation, including histological and radiological inflammation, a state with no or little risk of disease progression.

Improving disease symptoms used to be the goal in clinical practice and trials for many years. But treating patients' symptoms seemed to be insufficient, because patients experienced disease progression and bowel wall destruction.

More recently, mucosal healing, complete or partial healing, was suggested as treatment end point. Patients with mucosal healing have better long-term outcome, in terms of a decrease in active disease, reduction of long-term risk of corticosteroid usage [3, 29], and lower rates of hospitalizations and/or surgeries, compared to those without mucosal healing.

Trying to treat both clinical symptoms and inflammation, achieving deep remission [2] is a newer composite treatment end point. Patients achieving deep remission have better long-term outcome, compared to those only achieving clinical remission or only mucosal healing.

CTE and MRE are used in monitoring response to therapy in CD. There is a good correlation between endoscopic mucosal healing and CTE and MRE findings.

Both CTE and MRE have been shown to identify transmural radiological response with medical therapy.

CTE parameters that can decrease or even disappear during therapy include a decrease in bowel wall thickening and bowel wall enhancement, decrease in length of the disease, and decrease in dilatation of the vasa recta and perienteric fat stranding.

Several studies evaluated the effects of treatment on bowel wall lesions in active CD on CTE. Bruining et al. [30] evaluated, in a retrospective study several CTE abnormalities such as bowel wall enhancement and length of disease, and showed that 63% of patients had a significant radiologic therapy response to infliximab. In another retrospective study of 50 patients, Wu et al. [31] showed that some CTE abnormalities, like bowel wall thickening and mural hyperenhancement, decreased significantly after antibiotic and immunosuppressive therapy in correlation with clinical, endoscopic, pathologic, and laboratory findings.

An increasing number of studies show the utility of MRE in guiding treatment. MRE is a good tool for assessing response to therapy in CD patients.

The first study that evaluated the efficacy of MRE in therapy response was in 1999. The two MRE parameters that showed a significant decrease during therapy in that study were wall thickness and contrast enhancement of the bowel wall.

In a prospective study in 2014 of 48 patients with active CD, Ordàs et al. [1] evaluated changes of MRE parameters after corticosteroids or antitumor necrosis factor agents, at baseline and week 12, with ileocolonoscopy as reference standard.

Quantification of disease activity on endoscopy was done using the Crohn's Disease Endoscopic Index of Severity (CDEIS) and using the magnetic resonance index of activity (MaRIA) on MRE. This study demonstrated a good correlation between endoscopic achieved by mucosal healing and the resolution of mural and extramural findings on MRE, such as wall thickness, edema, contrast enhancement of the bowel wall, enlarged lymph nodes, fat stranding, and "comb sign."

Stoppino et al. [32] evaluated in a prospective study of 27 patients with moderate-to-severe CD MRE changes during treatment with anti-TNF, at baseline and week 26, in correlation with endoscopy, clinical evaluation, and C-reactive protein levels. They also found a good correlation between MaRIA score, endoscopic score, Simple Endoscopic Score for Crohn's Disease (SES-CD), and the clinical-biological markers. The diagnostic accuracy of MRE for predicting endoscopic healing/remission was comparable with the findings in the study of Ordas.

In another prospective study of 139 patients with CD in clinical and serological remission, Takenaka et al. evaluated the whole small bowel and also demonstrated that MRE is accurate in detecting changes after anti-TNF treatment [33].

CTE and MRE are able to detect changes to therapy, although in patients with endoscopic healing, there may remain CTE and MRE abnormalities, such as mild wall thickening, contrast enhancement, diffusion restriction, or others, which should be considered as residual findings.

5.5 Conclusion

CTE and MRE are the most adequate imaging tools for investigating the small bowel in patients with Crohn's disease. They are complementary to clinical and endoscopic information. These techniques can visualize the whole small bowel and can detect extraintestinal features if present. These cross-sectional imaging methods can show the presence, extent, and severity of CD, important information to guide patient's treatment.

Acknowledgment Special thanks to Mrs. Elly O'Connor.

References

1. Ordàs I, Rimola J, Rodriguez S, Paredes JM, Martinez-Pérez MJ, Blanc E, Arévalo JA, Aduna M, Andreu M, Radosevic A, Ramirez-Morros AM, Pino S, Gallego M, Jauregui-Amezaga A, Ricart E, Panés J. Accuracy of magnetic resonance enterography in assessing response to therapy and mucosal healing in patients with Crohn's disease. Gastroenterology. 2014;146: 374–82.
2. Colombel JF, Rutgeerts PJ, Sandborn WJ, Yang M, Camez A, Pollack PF, Thakkar RB, Robinson AM, Chen N, Mulani PM, Chao J. Adalimumab induces deep remission in patients with Crohn's disease. Clin Gastroenterol Hepatol. 2014;12:414–22.
3. Baert F, Moortgat L, Van Assche G, Caenepeel P, Vergauwe P, De Vos M, Stokkers P, Hommes D, Rutgeerts P, Vermeire S, D'Haens G. Mucosal healing predicts sustained clinical remission in patients with early-stage Crohn's disease. Gastroenterology. 2010;138:463–8.

4. Jauregui-Amezaga A, Rimola J, Ordàs I, Rodrigquez S, Ramirez-Morros A, Gallego M, Masamunt MC, Llach J, Gonzàlez-Suàrez B, Ricart E, Panés J. Value of endoscopy and MRI for predicting intestinal surgery in patients with Crohn's disease in the era of biologics. Gut. 2015;64:1397–402.
5. Huprich JE, Fletcher JG. CT enterography: principles, technique and utility in Crohn's disease. Eur J Radiol. 2009;69:393–7.
6. Leyendecker JR, Bloomfeld RS, DiSantis DJ, Waters GS, Mott R, Bechtold RE. MR enterography in management of patients with Crohn disease. Radiographics. 2009;29:1827–46.
7. Rimola J, Rodriguez S, Cabanas ML, Ayuso C, Panés J, Cuatrecasas M. MRI of Crohn's disease: from imaging to pathology. Abdom Imaging. 2012;37:387–96.
8. Tolan DJM, Greenhalgh R, Zealley IA, Halligan S, Taylor SA. MR enterographic manifestations of small bowel Crohn disease. Radiographics. 2010;30:367–84.
9. Bruining DH, Zimmermann EM, Loftus EV Jr, Sandborn WJ, Sauer CG, Strong SA; Society of Abdominal Radiology Crohn's Disease-Focused Panel. Consensus recommendations for evaluation, interpretation, and utilization of computed tomography and magnetic resonance enterography in patients with small bowel Crohn's disease. Gastroenterology. 2017. pii: S0016-5085(17)36658-1.
10. Hara EK, Swartz PG. CT enterography of Crohn's disease. Abdom Imaging. 2009;34:289–95.
11. Park MJ, Lim JS. Computed tomography enterography for evaluation of inflammatory bowel disease. Clin Endosc. 2013;46(4):327–66.
12. Takenaka K, Ohtsuka K, Kitazume Y, Nagahori M, Fujii T, Saito E, Naganuma M, Araki A, Watanabe M. Comparison of magnetic resonance and balloon enteroscopic examination of the small intestine in patients with Crohn's disease. Gastroenterology. 2014;147:334–42.
13. Takenaka K, Ohtsuka K, Kitazume Y, Nagahori M, Fujii T, Saito E, Fujioka T, Matsuoka K, Naganuma M, Watanabe M. Correlation of the endoscopic and magnetic resonance scoring systems in the deep small intestine in Crohn's disease. Inflamm Bowel Dis. 2015;2(8):1832–8.
14. Gale HI, Sharatz SM, Taphey M, Bradley WF, Nimkin K, Gee MS. Comparison of CT enterography and MR enterography imaging features of active Crohn disease in children and adolescents. Pediatr Radiol. 2017;47:1321–8.
15. Choi SH, Kim KW, Lee JY, Kim KJ, Lee JY, Kim KJ, Park SH. Diffusion-weighted magnetic resonance enterography for evaluating bowel inflammation in Crohn's disease: a systematic review and meta-analysis. Inflamm Bowel Dis. 2016;22(3):669–79.
16. Dohan A, Taylor S, Hoeffel C, Barret M, Allez M, Dautry R, Zappa M, Savoye-Collet C, Dray X, Boudiaf M, Reinhold C, Soyer P. J Magn Reson Imaging. 2016;44:1381–96.
17. Sato H, Tamura C, Narimatsu K, Shimizu M, Takajyo T, Yamashita M, Inoue Y, Ozaki H, Furuhashi H, Maruta K, Yasutake Y, Yoshikawa K, Watanabe C, Komoto S, Tomita K, Nagao S, Miura S, Shinmoto H, Hokari R. Magnetic resonance enterocolonography in detecting erosion and redness in intestinal mucosa of patients with Crohn's disease. J Gastroenterol Hepatol. 2015;30:667–73.
18. Oussalah A, Laurent V, Bruot O, Bressenot A, Bigard MA, Régent D, Peyrin-Biroulet L. Diffusion-weighted magnetic resonance without bowel preparation for detecting colonic inflammation in inflammatory bowel disease. Gut. 2010;59:1056–65.
19. Rimola J, Alvarez-Cofino A, Pérez-Jeldres T, Rodriguez S, Alfaro I, Ordàs I, Ricart E, Panés J. Increasing efficiency of MRE for diagnosis of Crohn's disease activity through proper sequence selection: a practical approach for clinical trials. Abdom Radiol. 2017;42(12):2783–91.
20. Allen BC, Leyendecker JR. MR enterography for assessment and management of small bowel Crohn disease. Radiol Clin North Am. 2014;52:799–810.
21. Li X, Mao R, Huang S, Sun C, Cao Q, Fang Z, Zhang Z, Huang L, Lin J, Chen Y, Rimola J, Rieder F, Chen M, Feng S, Li Z. Characterization of degree of intestinal fibrosis in patients with Crohn disease by using magnetization transfer MR imaging. Radiology. 2018;000:1–10.
22. Erden A, Ünal S, Akkaya HE, Onay M, Törüner M, Gençtürk ZB, Kartal AC. MR enterography in Crohn's disease complicated with enteroenteric fistula. Eur J Radiol. 2017;94:101–6.

23. Liu W, Liu J, Xiao W, Luo G. A diagnostic accuracy meta-analysis of CT and MRI for the evaluation of small bowel Crohn disease. Acad Radiol. 2017;24:1216–25.
24. Greenup AJ, Bressler B, Rosenfeld G. Medical imaging in small bowel Crohn's disease-computer tomography enterography, magnetic resonance enterography, and ultrasound: which one is the best for what? Inflamm Bowel Dis. 2016;22(5):1246–61.
25. Rimola J, Rodriguez S, Garcia-Bosch O, Ordas I, Ayala E, Aceituno M, Pellisé M, Ayuso C, Ricart E, Donoso L, Panés J. Magnetic resonance for assessment of disease activity and severity in ileocolonic Crohn's disease. Gut. 2009;58:1113–20.
26. Rimola J, Ordas I, Rodriguez S, Garcia-Bosch O, Aceituno M, Llach J, Ayuso C, Ricart E, Panés J. Magnetic resonance imaging for evaluation of Crohn's disease: validation of parameters of severity and quantitative index of activity. Inflamm Bowel Dis. 2011;17(8):1759–68.
27. Deepak P, Fletcher JG, Fidler JL, Barlow JM, Sheedy SP, Kolbe AB, Harmsen WS, Loftus EV, Hansel SL, Becker BD, Bruining DH. Radiological response is associated with better long-term outcomes and is a potential treatment target in patients with small bowel Crohn's disease. Am J Gastroenterol. 2016;111:997–1006.
28. Panaccione R, Colombel JF, Louis E, Peyrin-Biroulet L, Sandborn WJ. Evolving definitions of remission in Crohn's disease. Inflamm Bowel Dis. 2013;19(8):1645–53.
29. Reinink AR, Lee TC, Higgins PDR. Endoscopic mucosal healing predicts clinical outcomes in inflammatory bowel disease: a meta-analysis. Inflamm Bowel Dis. 2016;22:1859–69.
30. Bruining DH, Loftus EV, Ehman EC, Siddiki HA, Nguyen DL, Fidler JL, Huprich JE, Mandrekar JN, Harmsen WS, Sandborn WJ, Fletcher JG. Computed tomography enterography detects intestinal wall changes and effects of treatment in patients with Crohn's disease. Clin Gastroenterol Hepatol. 2011;9:679–83.
31. Wu YW, Tang YH, Hao NX, Tang CY, Miao F. Crohn's disease: CT enterography manifestations before and after treatment. Eur J Radiol. 2012;81:52–9.
32. Stoppino LP, Della Valle N, Rizzi S, Cleopazza E, Centola A, Iamele D, Bristogiannis C, Stoppino G, Vinci R, Macarini L. Magnetic resonance enterography changes after antibody to tumor necrosis factor (anti-TNF) alpha therapy in Crohn's disease: correlation with SES-CD and clinical-biological markers. BMC Med Imaging. 2016;16(1):37.
33. Takenaka K, Ohtsuka K, Kitazume Y, Matsuoka K, Nagahori M, Fujii T, Saito E, Kimura M, Fujioka T, Watanabe M. Utility of magnetic resonance enterography for small bowel endoscopic healing in patients with Crohn's disease. Am J Gastroenterol. 2017;464:1–12.

Functional Cross-Sectional Imaging Techniques in Crohn's Disease

6

Shankar Kumar, Nikhil Rao, and Stuart A. Taylor

Abstract

Imaging Crohn's disease poses significant challenges, particularly in precisely defining disease activity and monitoring the adequacy of therapeutic response. Observations based on the structure of the bowel and extra-enteric tissues are the mainstay of radiological interpretation. However, functional techniques which extract information beyond simple anatomy also show considerable promise and may contribute to individualised management of Crohn's disease patients. In this chapter, we summarise the importance and challenges posed by cross-sectional imaging of the bowel, focusing on magnetic resonance enterography (MRE). We then consider MR techniques that provide functional evaluation of the bowel over and above structure, including diffusion-weighted imaging (DWI), dynamic contrast-enhanced (DCE) imaging and assessment of bowel motility. Finally, we summarise the emerging data on the potential utility of positron emission tomography-magnet resonance imaging (PET-MRI) and positron emission tomography-computed tomography (PET-CT).

6.1 Introduction

Crohn's disease (CD), an idiopathic inflammatory bowel disorder, can affect any part of the gastrointestinal (GI) tract from the mouth to anus [1–4]. Classically, there is a discontinuous pattern of inflammation with diseased segments separated by areas of unaffected normal bowel, termed 'skip lesions'. Inflammation confined to the small bowel accounts for around 30% of cases, another 20% involve only the large bowel, with the remainder involving both the small bowel and colon [5].

S. Kumar · N. Rao · S. A. Taylor (✉)
Centre for Medical Imaging, University College London, London, UK
e-mail: stuart.taylor1@nhs.net

J. Rimola (ed.), *Cross-Sectional Imaging in Crohn's Disease*,
https://doi.org/10.1007/978-3-319-96586-4_6

The phenotype of CD is highly diverse ranging from superficial mucosal ulceration to penetrating transmural inflammation, inflammatory and fibrotic stricturing disease, fistula and abscess formation as well as a plethora of extra-intestinal manifestations [6–8]. These macroscopic bowel changes have been utilised in cross-sectional imaging to identify and quantify structural transmural damage and disease activity [9, 10].

At the microscopic level, there are many well-recognised features seen in CD including an increase in lamina propria cellularity, oedema, crypt irregularities, inflammatory cellular infiltrate, increased microvessel density, granuloma formation, lymphoid aggregates, changes in mural perfusion and fibrosis [11]. These histopathological changes underlie the utility of functional MRI techniques considered in this chapter.

In the following discussion, we will first briefly review the importance and challenges posed by imaging the structure of the bowel by cross-sectional imaging, with a focus on magnetic resonance enterography (MRE). This is covered in depth in other chapters. We will then consider MR techniques that provide functional evaluation of the bowel over and above structure, including diffusion-weighted imaging (DWI), dynamic contrast-enhanced (DCE) imaging and assessment of bowel motility. We then review emerging data on the potential utility of positron emission tomography-magnetic resonance imaging (PET-MRI) and positron emission tomography-computed tomography (PET-CT).

6.1.1 The Importance and Challenges of Enteric Assessment in Crohn's Disease

Accurate characterisation of disease status is fundamental to optimised patient management [1, 4]. This principle holds true across the full spectrum of CD care, from preoperative planning [12] to serial reassessment in patients receiving immune modulators [13]. The unpredictable, progressive and relapsing nature of the disease process requires periodic lifelong evaluation by radiological and endoscopic means [1, 8, 9, 14].

As discussed in other chapters, computed tomography (CT) enterography is a valuable technique, offering high-resolution imaging from a single breath-hold, and its high diagnostic yield is well described [15–18]. However, as detailed below, many functional cross-sectional imaging techniques such as assessment of motility or dynamic contrast enhancement require multiple image acquisitions at high temporal resolution, and given its associated radiation burden, the role of CT in functional bowel imaging is currently limited. This is particularly relevant in CD given that most patients present when young, with a peak incidence between 15 and 25 years [19]. Audits suggest approximately 10% of CD patients are exposed to potentially harmful doses of radiation [20], with over 15% acquiring a cumulative radiation dose that potentially increases their risk of cancer by over 7% [21]. Most of the data regarding functional imaging in CD has been acquired using radiation-free techniques, such as small bowel ultrasound and MRI, with an emphasis on the latter [22, 23].

6.1.2 Routine Applications of MRE

As discussed in previous chapters, MRE of the small bowel affords a high-tissue-contrast examination with multiplanar assessment of the abdomen and pelvis, without radiation exposure, and is increasingly used in clinical practice for assessment of disease activity, extent and complications and for monitoring response to therapy [24–26].

6.1.2.1 Technique

A full description of MRE technique and sequence selection is given in Chap. 5. In brief, enteric luminal distension is achieved by oral ingestion of a hyperosmolar, biphasic liquid [27]. This permits luminal distention for the duration of the examination with low signal intensity on T1-weighted sequences, permitting visualisation of small bowel enhancement and high signal intensity on T2-weighted sequences to identify bowel wall thickening. Sufficient luminal distension is vital as collapsed bowel can obscure or even mimic disease [23]. Modern scanners facilitate rapid acquisition of images, and a typical protocol may include fast spin echo (FSE) T2-weighted sequences (with and without fat saturation), steady-state free-precession gradient echo (SSFP GE) sequences without fat saturation and unenhanced and gadolinium-enhanced T1-weighted sequences. Typical sequences and an example of a good quality examination are illustrated in Fig. 6.1.

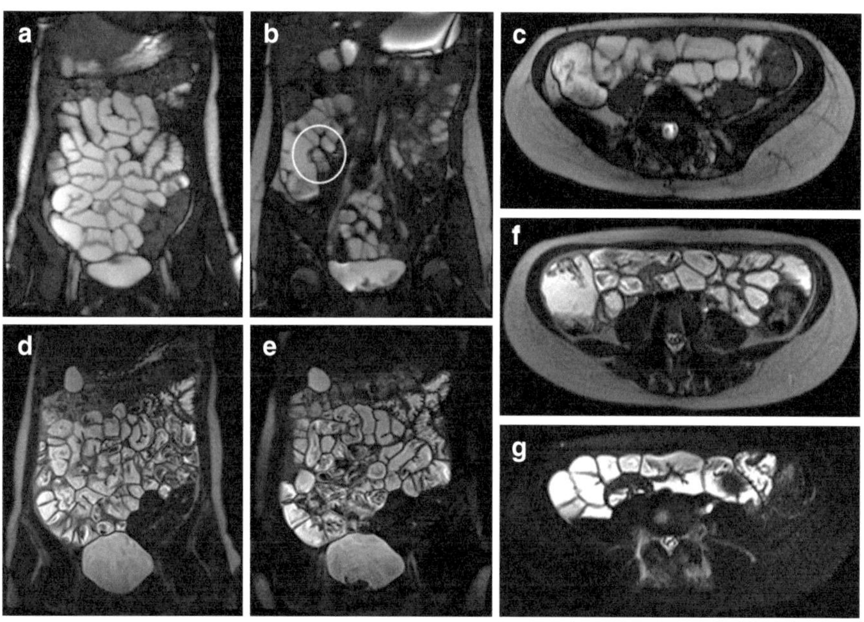

Fig. 6.1 MRI sequences in a standard MRE protocol; (**a**, **b**) Coronal steady-state free precession gradient echo (SSFP/Trufi) with good terminal ileum (white circle) distention. (**c**) Axial T2 Trufi. (**d**, **e**) Coronal and (**f**, **g**) axial T2 half-Fourier single-shot fast echo (HASTE) sequences with/without fat saturation, respectively

6.1.2.2 Interpretation of MRE

Routine clinical evaluation of MRE is based predominantly around the structure of the bowel and extra-enteric tissues. Morphological observations such as bowel wall thickness and the signal on T2- and post-contrast T1-weighted images form the bedrock of interpretation. As discussed fully in Chap. 10, various MRE activity scores have been developed and validated to aid phenotyping of disease activity in order to optimise delivery of target-directed therapy [28–30]. Examples include the magnetic resonance of activity (MaRIA) score (1.5 × bowel wall thickness (mm) × relative contrast enhancement (RCE) + 5 × oedema +10 × ulceration), the Crohn's Disease MRE Index (CDMI) (1.79 + 1.34 mural thickness score + 0.94 mural T2 signal score) [31] and its extended derivative, the magnetic resonance enterography global score (MEGS) [32]. MaRIA and CDMI are both reproducible between radiologists and highly sensitive for detecting and grading active CD [31, 33, 34]. At present, however, such scores are used mainly for research rather than in routine clinical practice.

Despite this emphasis on the structural information afforded by MRE, a range of functional techniques have been developed which further probe the underlying pathophysiology of CD, such as cellularity, vascular changes and peristaltic activity. Such techniques have potential as imaging biomarkers of inflammatory activity, both for disease phenotyping and therapeutic monitoring.

6.1.3 Diffusion-Weighted Magnetic Resonance Imaging (DWI)

6.1.3.1 Basic Principles Underpinning DWI

Diffusion of water molecules in biological tissues reflects the underlying architecture and histological properties [35]. Evaluating the diffusion of water molecules can therefore be exploited to model internal tissue structure and physiology. Changes in water motility occur as a result of interactions with cell membranes and macromolecules and changes in the tissue environment, which alter the Brownian motion and distribution of fluids. Pathological processes such as inflammation can disturb and alter the relative amount of diffusion occurring in the affected area. The differences in the diffusional properties between tissues can therefore be interrogated to reveal pathophysiological abnormalities and are the principles underpinning diffusion-weighted magnetic resonance imaging (DWI). Since its inception in 1985, DWI has evolved and is employed in many clinical applications, including neuroradiology, oncological and, more recently, in abdominal imaging [36].

Acquisition of DWI sequences utilises a T2-weighted fat-suppressed MR sequence in combination with a diffusion gradient, measured by a diffusion coefficient, the *b*-value [37]. As the *b*-value increases, there is a corresponding reduction in the signal in areas of free diffusion. Conversely, increasing the diffusion coefficient results in a slower decline of the signal in areas of restricted diffusion such as areas of increased cellularity. The acquired images undergo post-processing to extract parametric maps, and signal decay is modelled. Most commercial MR scanners make use of the mono-exponential fitting method, which offers a single parametric map referred to as the apparent diffusion coefficient (ADC) map [38]. By providing numerical values, ADC mapping permits quantification of diffusion restriction.

6.1.3.2 Application of DWI in Crohn's Disease

DWI has potential to provide information related to tissue perfusion, vascular leakage and water diffusion in CD. The inflammatory process in CD results in infiltration of the lamina propria and submucosal layer by lymphoid aggregates and inflammatory cells [11]. The resultant increase in cellularity, viscosity, granuloma formation and dilated lymphatics, all contribute to altered diffusion. Characteristic ulceration in CD is also associated with lymphoid aggregation, increased cell density and reduction of the extracellular space, all factors that can also restrict diffusion. This restricted diffusion manifests as high signal on high *b*-value images with corresponding low ADC values on ADC maps and is typically seen in active CD. However the exact microscopic basis for diffusion restriction in CD remains incompletely understood [28]. It is known, for example, that fibrosis also reduces the ADC, and bowel wall perfusion also likely influences the signal such that DWI does not simply reflect inflammatory activity [39]. Nevertheless, multiple studies using a range of reference standards have shown restricted diffusion in actively inflamed bowel segments [40–46].

DWI may have both clinical and research applications in CD. It has potential to improve MRE sensitivity for disease detection, and thereafter in assessing disease activity and response to therapeutic interventions. Finally, it may mitigate against the need to administer intravenous contrast.

6.1.3.3 Technical Aspects

Unlike routine MRI protocols which are now relatively well standardised, the technical parameters used for DWI remain heterogenous. Both 1.5-T and 3-T scanners can be used and both platforms appear adequate. Most studies use a single *b*-value or multiple *b*-values, with the highest ranging between 500 and 1000 s/mm^2, although there is a dearth of data pertaining to the optimal values [23, 28]. Feng et al., for example, reported that a high *b*-value of 1500 s/mm^2 was most suitable on their 3T platform [47].

Fasting is recommended between 2 and 6 h before the examination, to minimise peristalsis. Although it is feasible to perform DWI without antiperistaltic agents [48, 49], recent prospective data revealed that omission resulted in significantly reduced sensitivity for detecting bowel inflammation and underestimation of the extent of disease [50]. Adequate bowel distension, generally considered essential for a successful enterographic examination, is achieved by administering an oral contrast agent 45–60 min prior to image acquisition (see Chap. 5) [23]. Enteroclysis techniques, which require intestinal intubation under fluoroscopic guidance with associated radiation burden, have not yielded superior accuracy [51] and are therefore not recommended in routine protocols [23]. Only a handful of studies have reported on the fidelity of DWI for CD in the absence of an oral contrast agent, with varying success [42, 46, 52]. However, routine use of oral contrast is generally adopted, aiding standardisation and increasing consistency of results [28].

It is recommended that the patient is placed prone when performing DWI to improve distension of the bowel and to minimise both peristalsis and motion artefact, although superior accuracy compared to the supine position is yet to be formally demonstrated [53]. Some patients tolerate the prone position poorly, and there is an increased risk of vomiting, but otherwise this is the preferred posture for acquisition of images [23].

DW images are most often taken in the transverse plane as they are less prone to motion artefact than those acquired coronally. Navigator-trigger techniques or breath-holding can be used, with the advantage of reducing breathing motion artefact. However, these approaches increase acquisition time because images can only be obtained in certain respiratory phases, and potential reductions in signal-to-noise ratio can therefore impact on image quality. A signal averaging technique is therefore frequently employed, permitting the patient to breathe freely whilst images are acquired, increasing the signal-to-noise ratio. The use of free breathing protocols is therefore widespread [23].

Fat saturation or suppression techniques are important adjuncts to DWI to nullify the intrinsic high signal of mesenteric fat due to its short T1 relaxation time. The methods used are variable, but commonly a spoiler gradient is employed which saturates the fat signal, thereby suppressing it.

The DWI sequences performed at our institution are provided in Table 6.1.

6.1.3.4 Technical Limitations of DWI

Artefacts may be encountered when performing enteric DWI for several reasons. The required long acquisition times can result in motion artefacts. Gating techniques, faster imaging acquisition methods such as echo planar or parallel imaging, the use of antiperistaltic agents prior to the examination and novel motion compensation software algorithms are all strategies that can be employed to mitigate this [28]. The T2 shine-through effect is due to the intrinsic high signal of fluid within

Table 6.1 Typical sequences utilised at our institution, for DWI and motility imaging

Siemen symphony 1.5T		
Sequence	TE/TR	Slice thickness (mm)
T2 Trufi		
– Coronal 20 measures (CINE)	1.95/3.89	10
DWI axial b0, 600 free breathe	86/3600	5
ADC	86/3600	5
Philips Achieva 3T/motility sequences		
BTFE		
– Cine	1.8/3.7	6 × 5
– One image per second		
– Three to four blocks; six slices		
DWI axial b0–600 free breathe	51.4/2429	5
ADC	85/3600	5

Trufi true fast imaging with steady-state precession, *DWI* diffusion-weighted imaging, *ADC* apparent diffusion coefficient, *BTFE* balanced turbo field echo the bowel lumen and/or bowel wall and can give the appearance of restricted diffusion if only high *B* value images are reviewed. It is important to correlate with ADC maps where areas of restricted diffusion (low ADC) can be differentiated from areas of T2 shine-through (which exhibit a high ADC value). T2 shine-through effects can be minimised by using short echo times and high *b*-values.

6.1.3.5 Detecting Active Bowel Inflammation in Crohn's Disease

Many studies have explored the efficacy of simple qualitative evaluation of DWI to identify active CD, both in the small [29, 40, 42, 44, 45, 54–60] and large bowel [29, 40, 42, 44, 46, 55, 57–60]. They differ in their standard of reference for disease activity and variably employ conventional imaging, surgical findings, histopathology, endoscopy and MRE activity scores. They also differ in how they define abnormality on DWI imaging. Most compare the bowel wall signal to an internal reference such as adjacent normal bowel [40, 61] or the spleen [55, 62], for example. Some use a binary yes/no to define active disease [55] (Figs. 6.2 and 6.3), whilst others use grading systems from 1 to 4, for example [61]. The calculated ADC is also used by some studies, with heterogenicity in suggested cut-offs for active disease. Comparison across studies is therefore rather challenging.

Overall, the reported diagnostic performance of DWI is variable, with studies citing sensitivities and specificities between 68–100% and 51–100%, respectively. A systematic review and meta-analysis incorporating studies up to March 2015 concluded that although DWI sequences had good sensitivity in detecting inflammatory CD lesions, specificity was compromised [63]. The overall reported sensitivity and specificity were 92.9% (95% CI, 85.8–96.6%) and 91% (95% CI, 79.7–96.3%), respectively, but the authors noted significant heterogeneity across studies. Those studies not blinding readers to conventional sequences and/or using contrast-enhanced MRE as the standard of reference reported higher accuracy than studies not employing this methodology. Indeed, restricting the analysis to only studies using an endoscopic or a surgical reference standard resulted in an overall sensitivity for DWI of 84% with specificity of 73%. The relatively low specificity for DWI was underlined by a study by Kim et al. using a colonoscopic standard of reference [55]. Although adding DWI to conventional sequences increased sensitivity from 62 to 83% (mainly due to detection of subtle mucosal disease in the colon), specificity fell from 94% to just 60%. Most false positives occurred in the colorectum. The jejunum is another common site of DWI false positives, likely related in part to inadequate bowel distension (Figs. 6.4 and 6.5), and lymphoid hyperplasia of the terminal ileum can also be indistinguishable from active CD on DWI [64].

6.1.3.6 Quantitative Assessment of Inflammation

The ability of DWI to quantify the severity of bowel inflammation in CD has also been explored. Various groups have either used stand-alone ADC values on their own or combined DWI with morphological parameters from conventional MRE sequences. For example, the Clermont score comprises ADC values and several conventional MRE observations and is defined as $1.646 \times$ bowel thickness $-1.321 \times$ ADC $+ 5.613 \times$ oedema $+8.306 \times$ ulceration $+5.039$ [40]. The Clermont

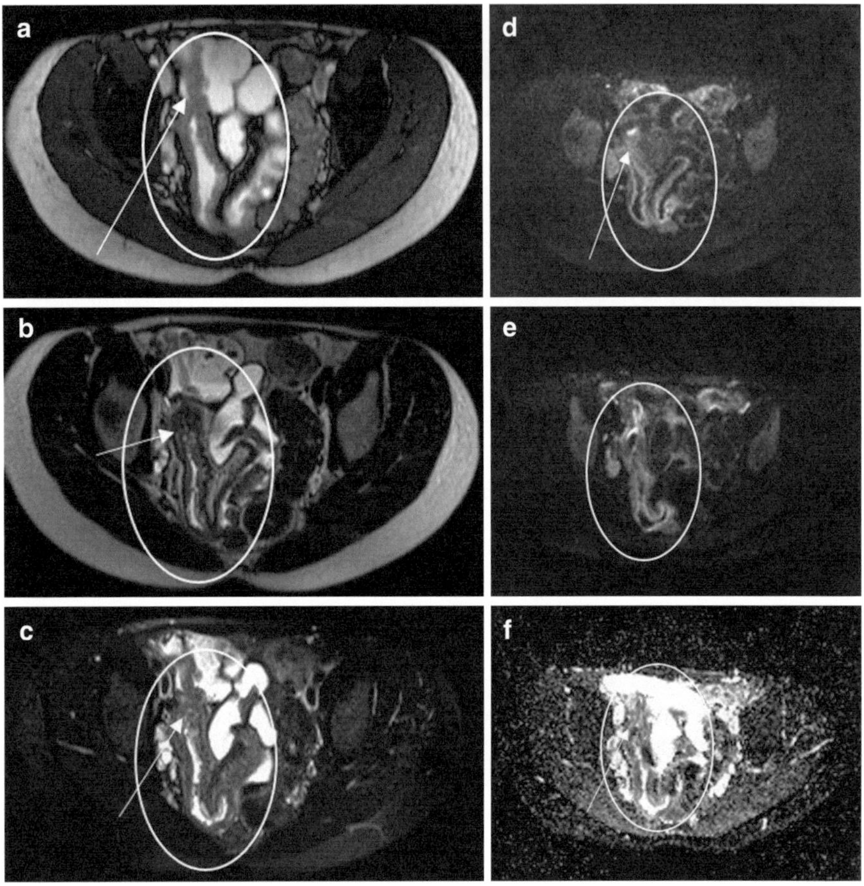

Fig. 6.2 Typical appearance of a long segment (>10 cm) of very active terminal ileal (white arrow and circled area) Crohn's on conventional sequences and DWI. Mural thickening, oedema and ulceration are shown on axial Trufi (**a**) and HASTE sequences without (**b**) and with (**c**) fat saturation. Axial DWI images show increased mucosal signal on (**d**, $B = 0$; and **e**, $B = 600$ s/mm^2). The ADC map (**f**) confirms a corresponding low signal area of restricted diffusion (white circles)

score is highly correlated with both the MaRIA [40, 45] and the Simplified Endoscopic Score for Crohn's Disease (SES-CD) [54, 65].

Again, given the lack of a single reference standard for Crohn's disease activity, authors have assessed DWI against a variety of reference standards, including MRE parameters [44, 66] and activity scores [40, 45, 54], endoscopic scores [54, 62, 67] and histopathological systems derived from surgical specimens [39]. In general, most studies report high correlation between DWI-/ADC- and MRE-derived activity scores and weak to moderate correlation against independent standard of reference such as endoscopy or histopathology. In study of 55 terminal ileum segments, Caruso et al. compared both the Clermont score and ADC to the reference standards of MaRIA and SES-CD. The correlation coefficients between Clermont and ADC

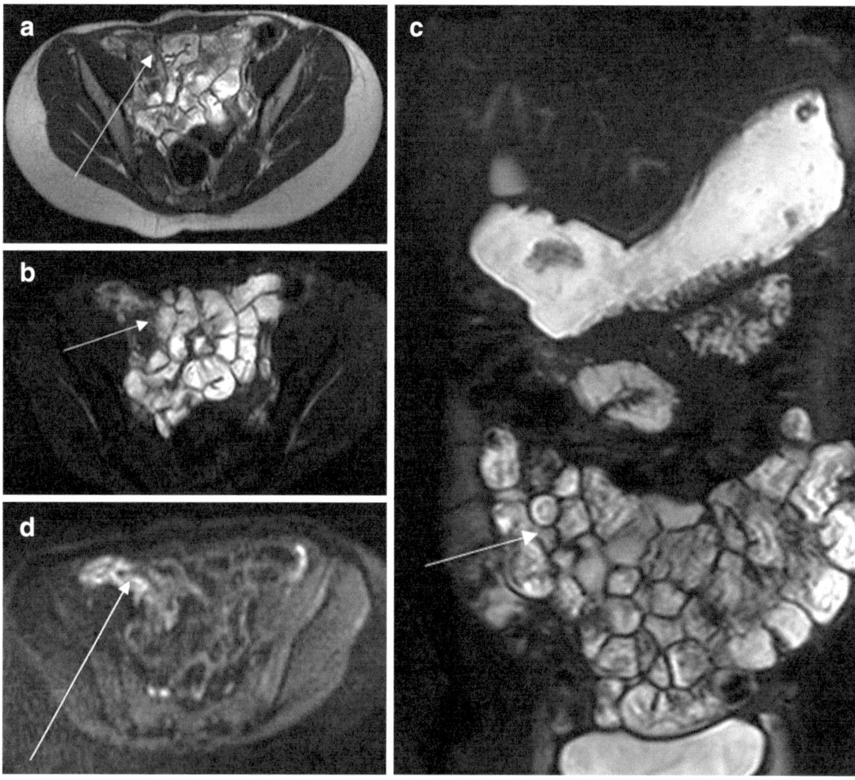

Fig. 6.3 Utility of diffusion-weighted imaging (DWI) in diagnosing terminal ileal Crohn's disease—The terminal ileum is under distended on the (**a**) axial T2 HASTE sequence, (**b**) axial HASTE fat saturated sequence and (**c**) coronal HASTE fat saturated sequence and so indeterminate for Crohn's disease involvement. (**d**) Axial DWI-weighted image (*B* value = 600 s/mm^2) shows abnormal increased linear high signal in the bowel wall suggestive of ileitis

with MaRIA were 0.91 and −0.80, respectively. When using the SES-CD score as the reference standard, the correlation coefficients with Clermont and ADC were 0.76 and −0.63, respectively [54]. Tielbeek et al. compared ADC to an acute inflammation scored derived from histopathological specimens in 27 bowel segments and reported a correlation coefficient of −0.33 [39]. Most recently, in a series of 39 terminal ileum segments, Seo et al. noted a correlation coefficient of 0.87, when comparing a semi-quantitative DWI score with endoscopy [62]. Pendsé et al. found that faecal calprotectin levels were significantly higher when DWI was abnormal in the small bowel and/or colon [14]. Of promise, abnormal DWI signal had a sensitivity of 83% for active CD based on faecal calprotectin as an independent reference standard, but specificity was disappointing at only 52%.

Although the literature suggests a relationship between DWI signal/ADC and the severity of bowel inflammation, the relationship is complex, and it is unlikely that a simple measure such as ADC can ever capture the complexity of the pathological

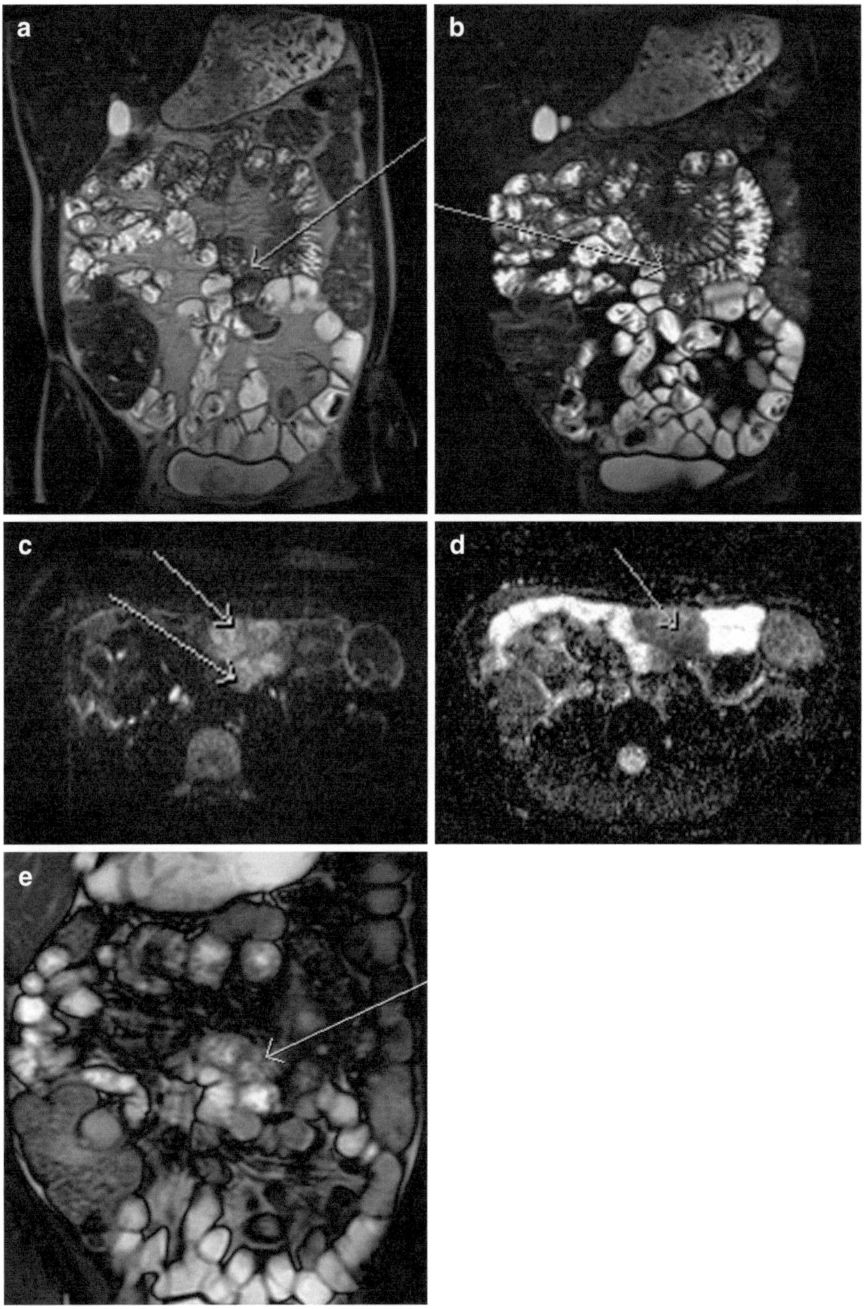

Fig. 6.4 False positive DWI, a common finding in under distended bowel, particularly in the jejunum (*arrows*), as seen on (**a**) coronal HASTE and with fat saturation (**b**). Apparent restricted diffusion as demonstrated on the DWI and corresponding ADC map ($B = 600$ s/mm^2) (**c**, **d**), but Cine Trufi T2 (**e**) sequence slabs show normal motility and distension of the corresponding bowel

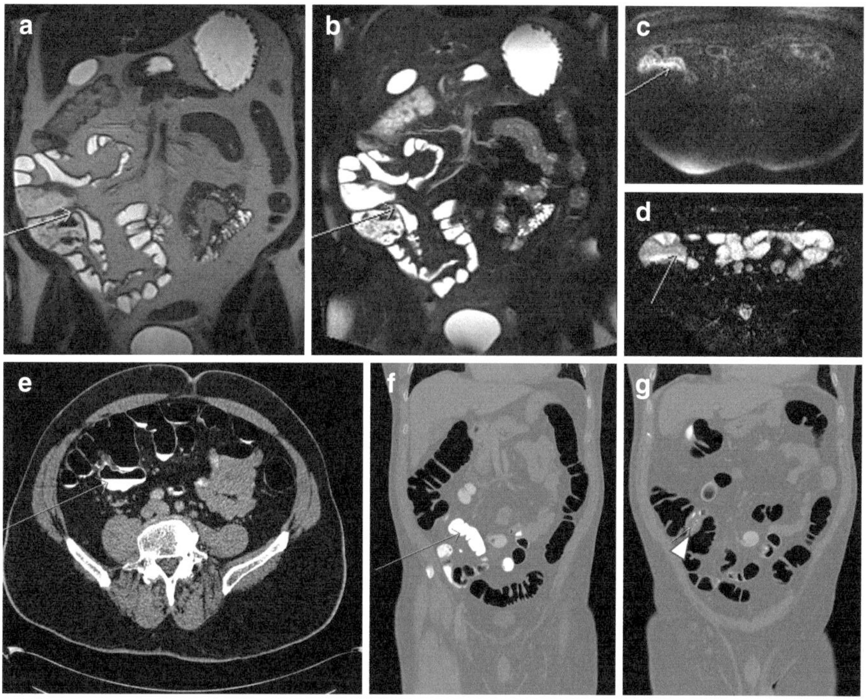

Fig. 6.5 False positive DWI, of the terminal ileum (*arrows*), which is partially collapsed as seen on coronal HASTE without (**a**) and with (**b**) fat saturation, although little in the way of mural thickening. Apparent restricted diffusion as demonstrated on the DWI (**c**) and corresponding ADC map ($B = 600$ s/mm^2) (**d**). The terminal ileum and ileocaecal valve (arrow head) were normal at CT colonography (**e**–**g**)

changes of CD. For example, Tielbeek et al. found that ADC correlated well with histopathologically quantified bowel wall fibrosis, but not with inflammation [39], a finding recently reproduced by Li et al. [58].

6.1.3.7 Treatment Response Evaluation

The utility of DWI to monitor the effects of therapy has been investigated by a few groups (Figs. 6.6 and 6.7). Bhatnagar et al. studied 23 patients monitored by DWI following treatment with tumour necrosis alpha antagonist therapy. They reported that ADC values increased significantly in clinical responders, with no significant change seen in patients who did not respond to immunosuppressive therapy [68]. Similarly, a Korean study of 18 patients found that endoscopic improvement of disease following medical therapy is associated with reduced mural diffusion restriction and higher ADC values [69]. Conversely, in a paediatric cohort, Dillman et al. reported that changes in ADC were just 58% sensitive and 52% specific for identifying response to tumour necrosis alpha antagonist therapy [70].

The utility of DWI to monitor treatment response therefore currently remains uncertain, and further research is required.

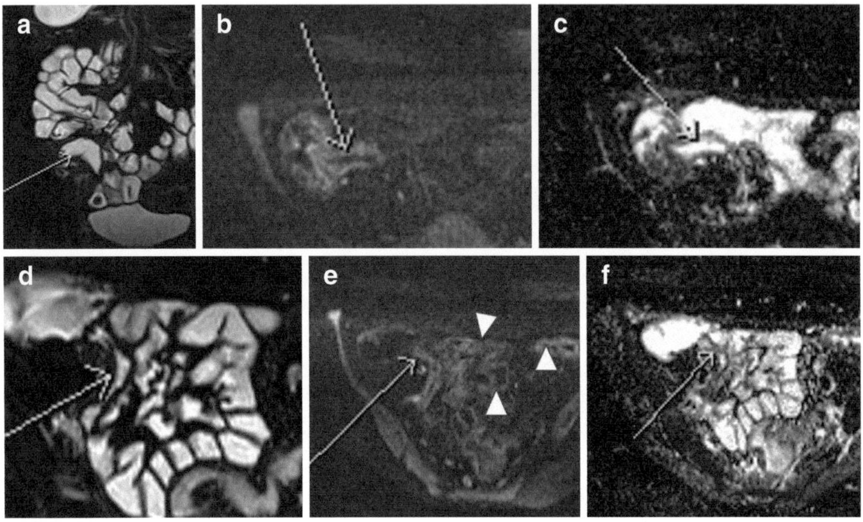

Fig. 6.6 Changes in DWI following treatment. There is a mildly thickened and active terminal ileal activity in a Crohn's patient, on coronal HASTE with fat saturation (**a**) and DWI (**b**), with mildly restricted diffusion on the ADC map (**c**). Subsequent follow-up on treatment 1 year later (**d**–**f**) still demonstrates some mild mural thickening, but the degree of restricted diffusion has improved to the level of adjacent/background bowel activity (arrows)

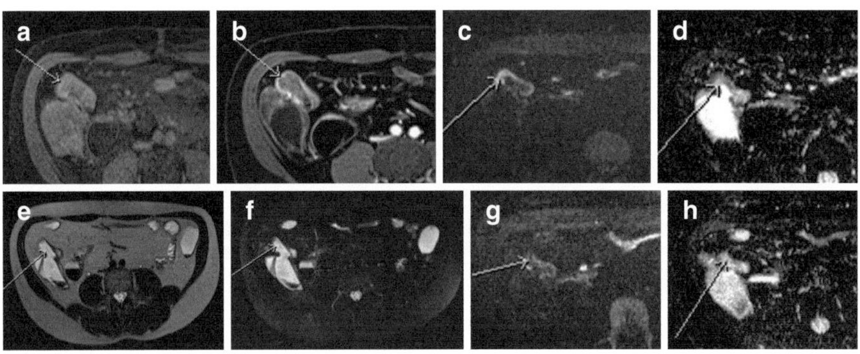

Fig. 6.7 Changes in DWI following treatment. There is mildly thickened and active neo-terminal ileal activity in a Crohn's patient with an ileo-colonic anastomosis shown on pre- (**a**) and post-contrast (**b**) fat saturation T1 sequences and DWI $B = 600$ s/mm^2) (**c**) with moderately restricted diffusion on the ADC map with (**d**). Subsequent follow-up 2 years later (**e**–**h**) demonstrates improved features with no mural oedema on fat sat HASTE sequence (**f**), reduced signal on DWI (**g**) and less restricted diffusion (**h**)

6.1.3.8 Replacement of IV Contrast Administration

Whilst administration of IV gadolinium remains part of standard MRE protocols (Fig. 6.8) [14], there are concerns about retention in the brain [71], and its use is occasionally contraindicated, such as in pregnancy, in individuals with documented allergy to contrast and in those with severely impaired renal function. There is therefore interest in replacing IV enhanced sequences with DWI.

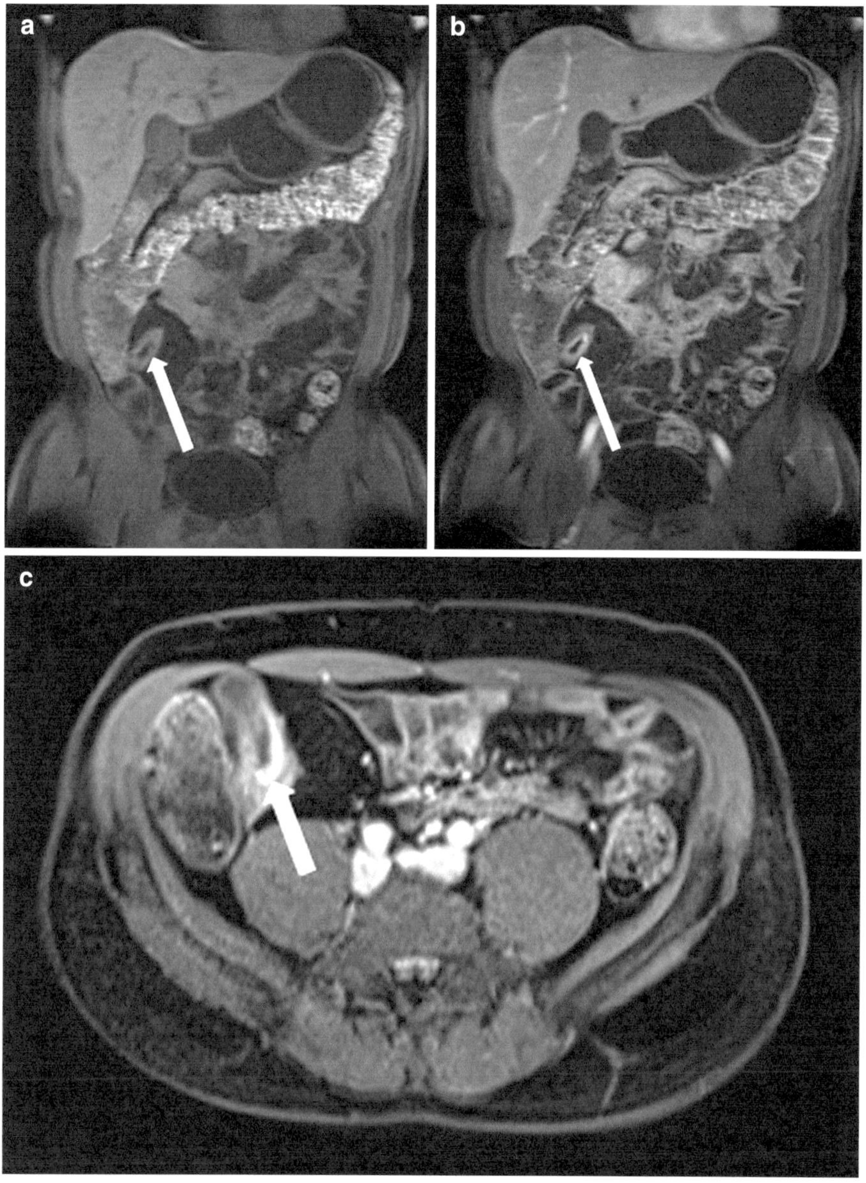

Fig. 6.8 Typical hyper-enhancement of active terminal ileal (*arrow*) Crohn's disease after IV gadolinium administration. (**a**) Pre-contrast coronal T1-weighted sequences with fat saturation. Post-contrast (**b**) coronal and (**c**) axial T1-weighted sequences with fat saturation show avid predominantly mucosal enhancement of the terminal ileum

In a non-inferiority study, Seo et al. reported that the diagnostic performance of T2-weighted images combined with DWI was equivalent to conventional MRE with T1 post IV contrast images [62]. It should be noted, however, that in this study the median CDEIS of the terminal ileum was 15.5, suggesting high prevalence of very active disease. Furthermore, of eight bowel segments with penetrating disease,

T2-weighted images combined with DWI missed a 2 cm sinus tract and incorrectly labelled 2.2 cm abscess as a phlegmon and a phlegmon as an entero-cutaneous fistula. All penetrating complications were correctly diagnosed using conventional MRE with T1 post IV contrast images.

In a paediatric cohort, Dubron et al. also reported that DWI was more accurate in detecting disease than contrast-enhanced imaging [72]. Notwithstanding these findings some mild lesions that are identifiable with contrast-enhanced MRE may be poorly detected on DWI [55, 62], In the author's institution, DWI has replaced T1-weighted post-contrast imaging in patients undergoing follow-up MRE for known CD, although this approach remains under investigation [28].

6.1.3.9 What Is the Clinical Role of DWI?

As discussed above, the evidence suggests that DWI used in combination with either T2-weighted sequences or T1-weighted sequences enhanced with gadolinium may improve the sensitivity of MRE for inflammatory lesions in CD, particularly if mild in severity [46, 55, 59]. However, there is an associated reduction in specificity. Furthermore, there may be no diagnostic advantage over conventional sequences for detecting more established inflammation, for example, when refining recruitment to clinical trials [29]. Recent consensus guidelines suggest that the use of DWI in routine MRE protocols remains optional [14] and, if used, DWI must always be used in conjunction with conventional MRE sequences.

At the author's institution, DWI is performed routinely and has replaced IV gadolinium in outpatient MRE follow-up of CD patients. We use it as an adjunct to conventional sequences and to help identify potential subtle disease, particularly in the colon, and provide a rapid overview of disease status. We do not use formal ADC measurements but subjectively evaluate DWI-weighted images as part of disease response evaluation, although priority is always placed on the findings on conventional sequences, notably T2-weighted images. We administer IV contrast in patients with known penetrating disease and in all hospital inpatients on the assumption that they are at higher risk of extra-enteric complications.

6.1.3.10 Summary

There is good evidence that active CD results in restricted diffusion within the bowel wall, although fibrosis has a similar effect. Sensitivity for subtle or early disease may be increased by adding DWI to conventional sequences, but specificity is reduced using this approach. DWI may have a role as an alternative to post IV gadolinium sequences in selected patients. The role of DWI in quantifying the severity of inflammation and assessing response to medical therapy requires further investigation before widespread clinical adoption.

6.1.4 Dynamic Contrast-Enhanced (DCE) Magnetic Resonance Perfusion Imaging

6.1.4.1 Basic Principles Underpinning DCE

The continual injury and regenerative process that occur in the bowel of CD patients lead to angiogenesis, driven by inflammation, hypoxia and the immune response [73]. This in turn results in an influx of inflammatory cells and greater expression of endothelial cells, inducing pro-inflammatory mechanisms and cytokine secretion. Indeed, the role of angiogenesis in CD has been extensively studied for over 50 years [74] and has been a therapeutic target [75]. Advanced functional imaging techniques able to estimate angiogenesis and quantify tissue haemodynamics have been invaluable in the study of tumour angiogenesis [76], with increasing interest in translating these methods to CD [77].

6.1.4.2 Applications of DCE-MRI in Crohn's Disease

It has long been established that there are marked macro and microscopic vascular changes in CD. Indeed, conventional angiography has been used in the past for diagnosis given the abnormal strictured and tortuous vessel anatomy adjacent to affected bowel [78], and in the era of cross-sectional imaging, engorgement of the vasa recta (comb sign) is often associated with active disease [9, 79]. Increased bowel wall enhancement following intravenous contrast administration on CT, MRE and ultrasound has been strongly linked to disease activity [80–82] and, as fully explored in Chap. 10, forms part of many imaging activity scores.

Studies have also shown that there is increased microvascular (MVL) density observed in intestinal tissue, which shows positive correlation with CD activity [83, 84]. However, the relationship between neoangiogensis and disease activity is complex. For example, it has been shown that bowel wall enhancement is correlated with the number of years post-diagnosis in patients with chronic disease and is also related to tissue hypoxia [85].

In conventional MRE and CTE protocols, images are acquired at one or two time points after administration of a single bolus of intravenous contrast (Chap. 5). These permit either qualitative or quantitative assessment of the relative enhancement of the bowel wall to look for the hyper enhancement associated with CD (Chap. 10). Dynamic contrast-enhanced imaging conversely acquires multiple images through the bowel with high spatial and temporal resolution to probe the local haemodynamics of the tissue.

Dynamic contrast-enhanced magnetic resonance imaging (DCE-MRI) in particular is an established technique that affords the opportunity to probe vascular structure and function. Applying DCE-MRI to CD to quantify physiological parameters related to enteric perfusion has the potential to provide greater insights into activity status than single-time point post-contrast images. Specifically, detailed functional data is derived from changes in blood flow and vascular permeability, as well as extravascular volumes. In this way, there is the potential to not only better differentiate active from inactive disease but also better grade the severity of disease. Furthermore, DCE imaging technique may play a role in furthering our understanding of the pathogenesis of CD and could help tailor therapy on a more individual basis.

6.1.4.3 Technical Aspects

A variety of pulse sequences are available for post-contrast for T1-weighted imaging including inversion recovery, gradient echo, fast spin echo and echo planar imaging. Gradient echo sequences (2D and 3D acquisitions) are frequently used as part of MRE protocols (Chap. 5) balancing signal to noise, bowel coverage, temporal resolution and production of artefacts. Prior to DCE, patient preparation is crucial; ingestion of oral contrast and administration of spasmolytic is routine.

DCE protocols acquire multiple images through the bowel wall often for several minutes (typically around 5–7 min) such that signal intensity can be plotted against time in the form of a time-intensity curve (TIC). The required temporal resolution is dependent on the planned analysis method. Simple evaluation of curve shape requires moderate temporal resolution achievable on most MRI scanners. The more quantitative analysis techniques described below require greater temporal resolution, and formal pharmacokinetic modelling requires resolutions at least below 5 seconds per volume [86] and ideally less; protocols achieving less than 1 second per volume are now possible [87]. It may be necessary to compromise on the volume of tissue interrogated as it is very difficult to image the whole small bowel volume with such high temporal resolution. Many workers therefore pre-identify the bowel section for DCE interrogation and limit the anatomical coverage. Thereafter, the problem of motion correction (peristalsis and breathing) must be overcome. Breath-hold protocols or those relying on respiratory triggering are often used, but this results in "gaps" in the data between acquisitions which may impact on quantitation particularly if a "gap" occurs around the crucial time of peak enhancement. Free-breathing protocols solve the problem of missing data, but motion correction is challenging. Various correction algorithms have been used including respiratory tracking (often of the diaphragm), volume preserving non-rigid registration, principal component registration [88], robust data decomposition registration [89] and more recently template-based registration [87]. Simpler approaches such as manually positioned ROIs whilst rejecting motion-corrupted images are also widely used in the literature.

Even when good quality motion-corrected DCE data is available, analysis is subject to many potential sources of error. Inhomogeneity in the B1 field is usually present across the imaged volume which impacts on quantitation. Thereafter, formal pharmacokinetic modelling requires calculation of the T1 relaxation time, knowledge of contrast volume/rate of administration, measurement or estimate of signal changes in nearby vascular structures (arterial input function), conversion TIC curves to concentration curves and finally, mathematical modelling.

It is of note that the linear relationship between iodine concentration and Hounsfield units means that DCE using CT is potentially more robust than MRI and is widely used in oncological imaging. However, as discussed above, the radiation doses associated with CT DCE protocols are currently generally viewed as prohibitive in young patients with non-neoplastic diseases, such as Crohn's disease.

A range of semi-quantitative measures can be derived from TIC, such as enhancement ratio, slope of enhancement and time to peak, which do not rely on complex mathematical models but nonetheless do require good-quality DCE data. These parameters can be rapidly derived but may not be reproducible for inter-patient comparison, particularly across different MRI platforms. Quantitative measures can be calculated based on the pharmacokinetics of the contrast agent as it traverses from the intravascular to extravascular-extracellular space, using mathematical models [90]. Most workers in CD have used the two-compartment Tofts model [90] from which commonly reported parameters are K^{trans} and V_e, measures of the volume transfer constant between intravascular space and extravascular-extracellular space and of extracellular extravascular volume per unit of volume tissue, respectively.

6.1.4.4 Detecting Active Bowel Inflammation in Crohn's Disease Semi-Quantitative DCE

As noted above, in general, increased bowel wall enhancement is a well-recognised finding suggesting active inflammation in CD [33, 91, 92] and is covered elsewhere in this volume. As well as facilitating quantitation of physiological parameters of perfusion, DCE-MRI allows the assessment of bowel wall enhancement with respect to time.

The literature concerning the use of DCE in CD is subject to the same variations in applied standards of reference than those described above for DWI. A range of reference standards have been used including endoscopy, surgical specimens, CRP and patient activity scores such as Crohn's Disease Activity Index (CDAI) and Harvey-Bradshaw Index (HBI). This complicates comparison between studies, but a defined association between semi-quantitative measures of DCE and disease activity has emerged.

Pupillo et al. reported a significant correlation between the peak of contrast uptake and severity of disease, assessed using the Crohn's Disease Activity Index (CDAI) [93]. They also noted a positive association between time to reach plateau and CDAI score, although statistical significance was not reached. In a 16-patient prospective cohort study, Del Vescovo et al. compared the enhancement kinetics of the bowel wall parietal layers with the degree of CD activity (measured using CDAI, CRP and histology) [94]. In patients with active disease, there was a rapid rise of mucosal-submucosal enhancement, with the peak reached 3 min after contrast administration. These changes were not seen in those with clinically inactive disease. These findings have been replicated in other studies comparing both diseased and normal bowel [95, 96] and clinically active versus dormant CD [97, 98]. Giusti et al., for example, reported that the maximum enhancement and slope of enhancement were significantly higher in patients with active disease defined using the CDAI, imaging patients over 6 min after the contrast injection [98]. Similarly, Rottgen et al. studied 26 patients with histologically proven CD and found that the slope of the contrast enhancement correlated significantly with local inflammation evaluated by ileocolonscopy [99]. Florie et al. used a free-breathing three axial slice protocol through abnormal bowel with a temporal resolution of 4–6 s over 2 min. They found a significant correlation between the bowel wall enhancement ratio, clinical grade of CD and the CDAI score [100]. More recently, in a prospective series of 33 CD patients, Ziech and co-workers described a significantly greater maximum enhancement in both severe and mild CD when compared to normal bowel mucosa [101], and using surgical resection specimens, Tielbeek et al. reported a positive correlation between the T1 ratio, maximum enhancement and initial slope of increase and a histological transmural acute inflammation score (AIS) [39].

6.1.4.5 Quantitative Assessment of Bowel Inflammation

Promising data from semi-quantitative analysis of DCE as described above has generated great interest in the possible opportunities afforded by DCE-MRI. Utilising quantitative, rather than semi-quantitative, measures could provide functional data directly relating to physiological parameters of vascular perfusion in the bowel wall of CD patients. An additional benefit is that comparisons could potentially be made between patients across different scanners, if the correct QA systems are in place. However, despite this, relatively few studies have used formal pharmacokinetic modelling in CD.

A pilot study of 51 bowel segments (19 with inflammation) in 11 patients that used endoscopic and surgical standards of reference tested a DCE protocol with a temporal resolution of 5–12 s in which image acquisition was over 5–7 min [96]. Inflamed bowel had greater K^{trans} and V_e values than normal bowel. Similarly, in a study of 21 patients principally designed to compare methods for estimating the arterial input function, van Schie et al. reported a good correlation between K^{trans} and CDEIS of 0.73 ($p < 0.001$) [102].

Zu et al. studied 32 patients with CD and 18 healthy volunteers and compared DCE parameters against the CRP as a marker of disease activity [103]. K^{trans}, K_{ep} and V_e were all higher in the CD patients than controls, and both K^{trans} and V_e were correlated to CRP ($r = 0.72$, $p < 0.001$, and $r = 0.53$, $p = 0.002$), respectively.

However, a study by Taylor et al. did not corroborate the link between disease activity and quantitative DCE parameters. They found no correlation between quantitative parameters and clinical nor histological markers of inflammatory CD using surgical resection specimens [85].

These conflicting data highlight the need for further studies to further explore and clarify the utility of these quantitative measures.

6.1.4.6 Treatment Response Evaluation

There are emerging data assessing the efficacy of DCE-MRI to evaluate response to therapy in CD. In a study of 27 patients who received tumour necrosis factor alpha antagonist therapy and followed up by DCE-MRI, Bhatnagar et al. found a significant difference in a number of quantitative measures in treatment responders, not seen in those who did not exhibit a clinical response to treatment [68]. Specifically K^{trans} and slope of enhancement changed significantly in clinical responders but not in nonresponders.

Similarly, Zhu and colleagues studied 22 CD patients treated by faecal microbiota transplantation (FMT) and found a significant difference in the K^{trans} and blood volume, measured by DCE-MRI in those demonstrating a clinical response [103].

6.1.4.7 What Is the Clinical Role of DCE-MRI in Crohn's Disease?

It is known that enteric contrast enhancement is related to CD activity. Simple qualitative grading or signal intensity measurements of a single post-contrast dataset are effective and widely used in clinical practice. DCE holds promise as a more quantitative method to assess abnormal perfusion associated with CD, but protocols are relatively complex, requiring high temporal resolution over long periods, usually with post-processing motion correction. Analysis is prone to error and requires relatively complex modelling. Whilst there is good date suggesting semi-quantitative parameters are related to disease activity, it is not clear if these add anything to the simpler evaluation of enhancement on a single-time point post-contrast dataset performed as part of routine MRE protocols. Thus, DCE is rarely used clinically and is limited to mainly a research setting. Similarly, formal quantitative modelling of DCE shows promise as a biomarker of disease activity and marker of therapeutic response but is to date mainly a research tool. Overall DCE is not currently considered a mandatory component of MRE protocols but can provide useful quantitative measures of contrast enhancement and can be used as an experimental adjunct [14].

6.1.4.8 Summary

There are profound vascular changes related to CD. Whilst these are driven by several factors, data suggests there is a link with inflammatory activity. There is a reasonable evidence base linking semi-quantitative measures of contrast enhancement with inflammatory burden in CD. Notwithstanding, quantitative measures that directly measure physiological parameters facilitate more robust comparisons between patients. Future studies are needed to clarify the utility of quantitative measures and further explore the role of DCE-MRI as a means of assessing therapeutic response.

6.1.5 Cine-MRE

Traditional fluoroscopic studies have long demonstrated altered motility in bowel segments affected by inflammation in CD. However, the clinical utility of this observation has until recently received little attention as this modality imparts ionising radiation and lacks methods of quantification, and use has generally fallen out of favour [104]. The ability of MRI to safely capture bowel motility has however rekindled interest.

6.1.5.1 Application of Cine MRE in Crohn's Disease

The bowel wall contains smooth muscle cells which drive peristalsis through coordinated contraction of the circular muscle layer. This is controlled by the plexus myentericus of Auerbach which has also been described as the "brain of the gut". There are broadly two types of contractility with postprandial actions and fasting activity. Postprandial actions such as peristalsis and segmentation occur after ingesting food to mix it and aid its absorption. Fasted contractility such as the migrating motor complex occurs between meals and is thought to be for maintaining bowel health and function.

The underlying mechanisms for reduced motility in Crohn's affected bowel are multifactorial, but inflammatory and fibrotic infiltration, neuritis within the bowel wall and systemic effects of the inflammatory burden mediated via hormonal and neuronal pathways all likely play a role.

6.1.5.2 Technical Aspects

Hardware and software advances mean that bowel motility can be captured as part of routine MRE protocols, using standard MRI platforms [105]. The bowel is prepared using a standard oral contrast agent (Chap. 5), and this contrast volume stimulates bowel motility. Most commonly, motility is usually captured using 2D fast "cine" sequence such as T2-weighted steady-state free precession (SSFP) or echo-planar cine sequences. Data suggests temporal resolution of one image per second for at least 15 s during a breath-hold is adequate to meaningfully capture segmental bowel motility [106]. 3D sequences remain under investigation, as do techniques based on the insertion of "taglines" into the image acquisition to measure motility over time [107].

Images are typically acquired as a coronal slab (usually 1 cm thick) during a breath-hold, which is repeated after moving the position of the slab to cover the whole small bowel volume.

The recent advances in MR small bowel motility imaging have mainly been due to the development of post-processing software solutions that can reliably quantify motility; visual inspection lacks reproductivity, and manual measurements are prohibitively time-consuming for clinical use [108].

There are various software solutions available such as semiautomated bowel lumen calibre measurement [109] and displacement mapping [110] which uses registration techniques to produce a surrogate of motility based on modelling of intensity changes over time caused by bowel motility and movement of luminal content. One commonly applied technique uses the Jacobian determinant calculated from the deformation fields in a manually drawn region of interest over the bowel. In a 2D image, this represents the area change that each individual pixel in an image undergoes when being transformed to the equivalent pixel in a reference image (Fig. 6.9) [110].

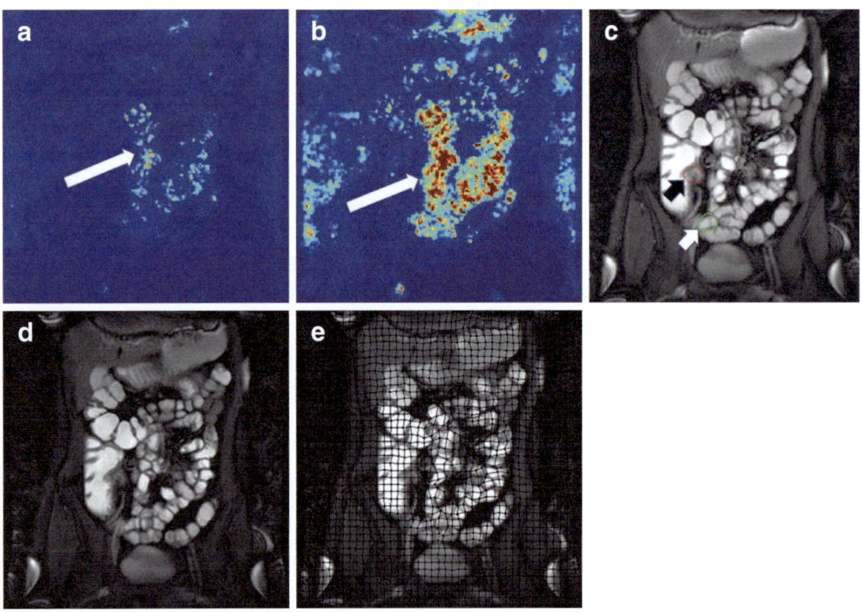

Fig. 6.9 Quantitative evaluation of dynamic motility data. A dynamic series has been processed with a specialised non-rigid registration algorithm (GIQuant, Motilent, Ford, UK) to produce a motility map (**a**, **b** white arrows) with areas of high motility attracting a high motility score [**c** regions of interest (ROI) around terminal ileum (black arrow) motility score is 0.055 vs. small bowel (white arrow) score of 0.343]. The motility score is based on the size of the deformation field produced by each of the image time points in the series to the registration target image or reference (**d**). A visual representation of the deformation fields can be seen in (**e**). Areas of high motility will undergo greater deformation over time

The motility sequence parameters performed at our institution are provided in Table 6.1.

6.1.5.3 Detecting Active Bowel Inflammation in Crohn's Disease

Most work researching the use of motility imaging in Crohn's disease has investigated the link between reduced segmental motility and the underlying inflammatory burden, although Froehlich et al. tested the additional diagnostic impact of motility sequences over conventional MRE protocols [111]. In a study of 40 patients with histologically proven CD, cine MRE was able to identify 35 more CD-specific findings than conventional MRE alone ($p = 0.0007$).

Menys et al. studied 28 patients with CD, all undergoing cine MRE with true fast imaging, steady-state precession (true FISP) sequences [112]. A software-quantified motility index was calculated from the terminal ileum and inflammatory activity measured using the endoscopic acute inflammation score (eAIS) based on histological analysis of endoscopic biopsies. Quantified terminal ileum motility correlated negatively with both eAIS ($r = -0.52$, $p = 0.005$) and an MR activity index of CD incorporating recognised parameters including T2 signal intensity and wall thickness ($r = -0.7$, $p < 0.001$). Cullman et al. reported similar findings in a cohort of 43 patients, although also reported that reduction in motility was associated with chronic as well as acute histological changes in the small bowel [113].

Hahnemann et al. reported that bowel segments with stigmata of CD on MRE had lower motility than non-affected bowel [114], a finding reproduced by Akerman and colleagues in 127 nonselected patients undergoing MRE [115]. Motility of the terminal ileum was significantly lower when compared to healthy controls ($p = 0.018$), and subgroup analysis revealed that this difference persisted in patients with CD limited to the small bowel ($p = 0.002$).

The effect of treatment on motility has also been investigated [116]. In a cohort of 46 patients undergoing anti-TNFα therapy, responders (defined by change in physician global assessment, HBI, CRP and MRI activity score) had significantly greater improvement in segmental motility than their nonresponding counterparts ($p < 0.001$). Improved MRI-measured motility was 93.1% sensitive (95% CI: 78.0–98.1%) and 76.5% specific (95% CI: 52.7–90.4%) for anti-TNFα response. Importantly, improvement in motility occurred as early as 12 weeks, suggesting motility may improve before some structural markers of activity on MRE.

Crohn's disease patients often report persistent symptoms such as abdominal pain, bloating and diarrhoea, even when the disease is in apparent remission with little or no inflammatory activity. MRI has been used to measure motility in apparently healthy bowel not directly affected by Crohn's disease in order to investigate whether aberrant motility underlies such persistent symptoms.

In a prospective study of 53 CD patients, Menys et al. demonstrated a significant negative correlation between motility variance (i.e. how much variation there was in the motility of apparently normal small bowel) and patient self-reported well-being ($r = -0.4$, $p = 0.003$), pain ($r = -0.27$, $p = 0.05$) and diarrhoea ($r = -0.4$, $p = 0.0025$) [117]. There was also a negative correlation with calprotectin, a marker of activity ($r = -0.33$, $p = 0.015$), a finding also reported by Bickelhaupt et al. who found contraction frequency was inversely correlated to calprotectin levels [118]. These data suggest subclinical inflammation may have a systemic effect on general gut motility likely via hormonal and/or neuronal pathway and is linked to persistent abdominal symptoms.

6.1.5.4 What Is the Clinical Role of Cine MRI?

There is increasing evidence that reduced segmental small bowel motility is correlated to inflammatory activity in Crohn's disease and that motility improves with successful treatment. However, like DWI and DCE-MRI, consensus recommendations state that motility sequences are optional as part of MRE protocols [14]. In the author's institution, motility sequences are acquired routinely and analysed subjectively by radiologists to help grade activity in stricturing disease as an adjunct to standard morphological criteria and to help confirm normality of poorly distended bowel loops (Figs. 6.10 and 6.11).

6.1.5.5 Summary

The link between MRI quantified small bowel motility, inflammatory burden and treatment response is being established. However, multicentre studies are currently underway to further test this association and to confirm whether it is robust across a range of patients, MRI scanners and radiological observers. Further mechanistic research is also underway investigating the use of MRI in quantifying aberrant bowel motility in symptomatic Crohn's disease patients. Small bowel motility is an exciting technique which will likely play an increasing role in the imaging of Crohn's disease.

6.1.5.6 PET/MRI and PET/CT

There has been interest in applying hybrid imaging techniques, combining positron emission tomography (PET) with MRI or CT to CD, inspired by the successes in other clinical settings such as oncology [119]. A commonly used radiotracer in PET imaging, 18F-fluorodeoxyglucose (18F-FDG), permeates cell membranes via specific

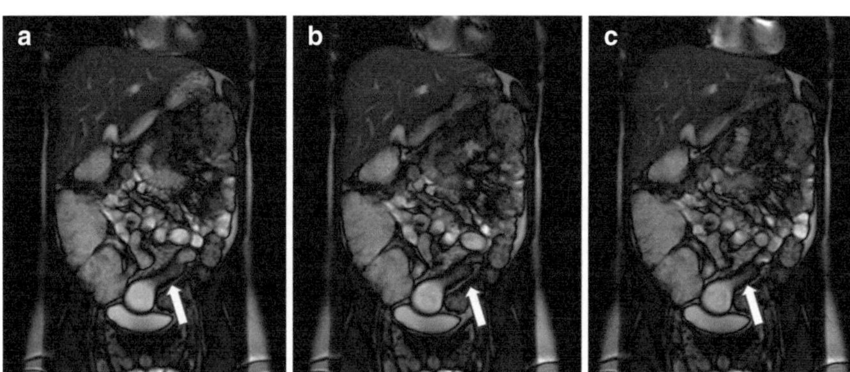

Fig. 6.10 Absent motility in a chronic Crohn's disease stricture (*arrow*). (**a**–**c**) Sample images from a cine motility Trufi sequences through the stricture showing no peristaltic movement

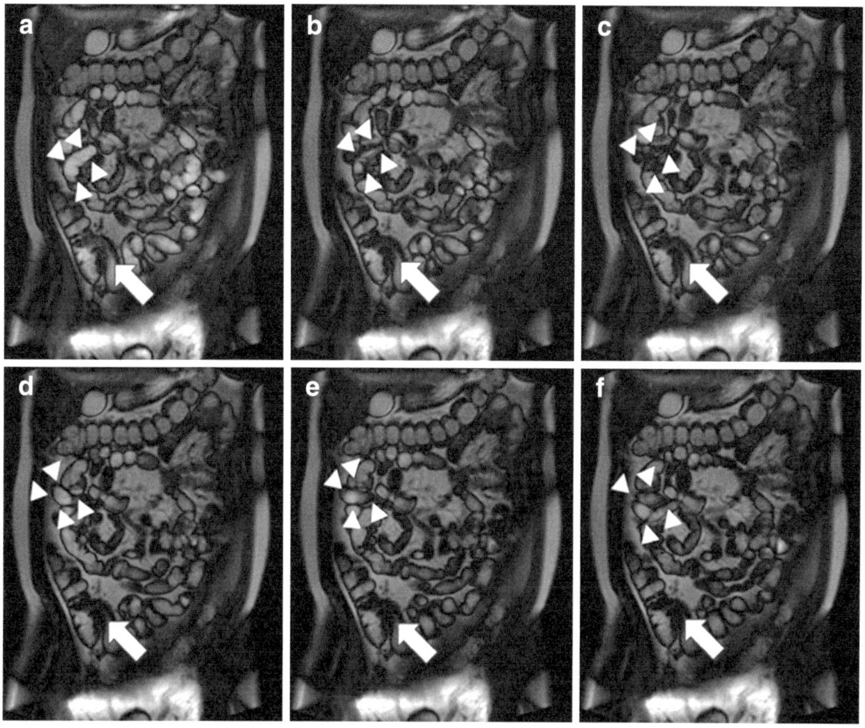

Fig. 6.11 Absent motility in a terminal ileal Crohn's disease. (**a**–**f**) Sequential Trufi CINE images of the terminal ileum (*arrow*) show a short segment of terminal ileal disease with minimal motility in comparison with normal small bowel (arrow heads)

channel proteins and tends to accumulate in regions where there is high glucose uptake and utilisation, for example, in inflammatory cells [120]. Indeed, 18F-FDG uptake has been shown to correlate with active inflammation in CD [121]. Hybrid imaging combining PET with CT is well described, and several studies have shown its ability to detect active CD in the small and large bowel [122, 123], but the radiation burden that it confers is a major limitation. In a prospective study of 28 patients using PET-CT, there was significantly greater radiotracer uptake in areas of active CD when compared to normal bowel wall segments [124]. Saboury et al. correlated FDG PET parameters with an endoscopic score of disease activity in 22 patients and found significant correlation between CDEIS and standardised uptake value (SUV) max [125]. Using MRI as a standard of reference, Russo et al. investigated PET-CT for treatment follow-up [126]. Thirteen patients underwent PET-CT and MRI before and 12 weeks after starting antitumour necrosis factor-alpha therapy. There were significantly greater falls in SUV_{max} in those who responded than in those who did not.

The possibility of amalgamating the anatomical detail afforded by MR with the detailed physiological molecular data that PET provides, thereby minimising radiation exposure, is highly appealing. To date, few studies have evaluated the clinical utility of PET/MRI, and whether it leads to an incremental benefit over performing these studies alone remains unclear [127]. Pellino et al. compared the accuracy and clinical impact of PET/CT with PET/MRI and MR alone, in a prospective study of 28 CD patients [128]. Despite all three modalities being equally accurate in detecting active disease, PET/MRI was more accurate than PET/CT in detecting fibrotic and extra-luminal disease. The latter translated to significantly reduced operating times, with a direct impact on clinical outcome. In a retrospective study of 19 CD patients, the same research group evaluated PET/MRI to discern fibrotic and inflammatory stricturing disease using the gold standard of histology from surgical specimens [129]. The authors found that the multiplication of the PET/MRI biomarkers of signal intensity (SI), PET maximum standardised uptake value (SUV_{Max}) and ADC was significantly different between the fibrosis only, active inflammation and fibrosis with active inflammation groups. Their observation that PET/MRI could differentiate between fibrotic disease with minimal inflammation and fibrosis with a high associated inflammatory burden could be of considerable practical importance, as these clinical entities are managed in different ways [130]. The findings were, however, at odds to those of a previous study which found no difference in the ability of PET, MRI or US to classify the nature of Crohn's strictures [131].

6.1.5.7 Summary

Undoubtedly, more studies are needed to assess the role of PET/MRI in CD. Differentiating inflammatory from fibrotic strictures is a promising potential application accepting that PET does expose patients to radiation. Furthermore, combining the morphological detail of MRI, along with advanced sequences like DWI and DCE-MRI and the metabolic data from PET, could offer exciting means of acquiring detailed functional data in CD.

6.2 Chapter Summary

Routine clinical evaluation of MRE is based predominantly around the structure of the bowel and extra-enteric tissues. However, techniques capturing the functional abnormalities in the bowel show considerable promise, particularly DWI and motility imaging. PET MRI remains under active investigation. Perhaps the most promising potential role of functional techniques is in the assessment of disease activity and therapeutic monitoring. More research is needed, for example, to confirm the reproducibility of functional techniques across institutions and to confirm the diagnostic benefit over standard MRI evaluation, but it seems likely that they will play an increasing role in the evaluation of CD.

References

1. Farmer RG, Whelan G, Fazio VW. Long-term follow-up of patients with Crohn's disease. Relationship between the clinical pattern and prognosis. Gastroenterology. 1985;88:1818–25.
2. Sands BE. From symptom to diagnosis: clinical distinctions among various forms of intestinal inflammation. Gastroenterology. 2004;126:1518–32.

3. Podolsky DK. Inflammatory bowel disease. N Engl J Med. 2002;347:417–29.
4. Van Assche G, Dignass A, Panes J, et al. The second European evidence-based consensus on the diagnosis and management of Crohn's disease: definitions and diagnosis. J Crohns Colitis. 2010;4:7–27.
5. Farmer RG, Hawk WA, Turnbull RB Jr. Clinical patterns in Crohn's disease: a statistical study of 615 cases. Gastroenterology. 1975;68:627–35.
6. Fiocchi C. Inflammatory bowel disease: etiology and pathogenesis. Gastroenterology. 1998;115:182–205.
7. Louis E, Collard A, Oger AF, Degroote E, Aboul Nasr El Yafi FA, Belaiche J. Behaviour of Crohn's disease according to the Vienna classification: changing pattern over the course of the disease. Gut. 2001;49:777–82.
8. Lichtenstein GR, Hanauer SB, Sandborn WJ, Practice Parameters Committee of American College of Gastroenterology. Management of Crohn's disease in adults. Am J Gastroenterol. 2009;104:465–83. quiz 4, 84
9. Benitez JM, Meuwis MA, Reenaers C, Van Kemseke C, Meunier P, Louis E. Role of endoscopy, cross-sectional imaging and biomarkers in Crohn's disease monitoring. Gut. 2013;62:1806–16.
10. Pariente B, Peyrin-Biroulet L, Cohen L, Zagdanski AM, Colombel JF. Gastroenterology review and perspective: the role of cross-sectional imaging in evaluating bowel damage in Crohn disease. AJR Am J Roentgenol. 2011;197:42–9.
11. Magro F, Langner C, Driessen A, et al. European consensus on the histopathology of inflammatory bowel disease. J Crohns Colitis. 2013;7:827–51.
12. Otterson MF, Lundeen SJ, Spinelli KS, et al. Radiographic underestimation of small bowel stricturing Crohn's disease: a comparison with surgical findings. Surgery. 2004;136:854–60.
13. Travis SP, Stange EF, Lemann M, et al. European evidence based consensus on the diagnosis and management of Crohn's disease: current management. Gut. 2006;55(Suppl 1):i16–35.
14. Taylor SA, Avni F, Cronin CG, et al. The first joint ESGAR/ESPR consensus statement on the technical performance of cross-sectional small bowel and colonic imaging. Eur Radiol. 2017;27:2570–82.
15. Hara AK, Leighton JA, Heigh RI, et al. Crohn disease of the small bowel: preliminary comparison among CT enterography, capsule endoscopy, small-bowel follow-through, and ileoscopy. Radiology. 2006;238:128–34.
16. Lee SS, Ha HK, Yang SK, et al. CT of prominent pericolic or perienteric vasculature in patients with Crohn's disease: correlation with clinical disease activity and findings on barium studies. AJR Am J Roentgenol. 2002;179:1029–36.
17. Siddiki HA, Fidler JL, Fletcher JG, et al. Prospective comparison of state-of-the-art MR enterography and CT enterography in small-bowel Crohn's disease. AJR Am J Roentgenol. 2009;193:113–21.
18. Higgins PD, Caoili E, Zimmermann M, et al. Computed tomographic enterography adds information to clinical management in small bowel Crohn's disease. Inflamm Bowel Dis. 2007;13:262–8.
19. Cosnes J, Gower-Rousseau C, Seksik P, Cortot A. Epidemiology and natural history of inflammatory bowel diseases. Gastroenterology. 2011;140:1785–94.
20. Chatu S, Subramanian V, Pollok RC. Meta-analysis: diagnostic medical radiation exposure in inflammatory bowel disease. Aliment Pharmacol Ther. 2012;35:529–39.
21. Desmond AN, O'Regan K, Curran C, et al. Crohn's disease: factors associated with exposure to high levels of diagnostic radiation. Gut. 2008;57:1524–9.
22. Allen PB, De Cruz P, Lee WK, Taylor S, Desmond PV, Kamm MA. Noninvasive imaging of the small bowel in Crohn's disease: the final frontier. Inflamm Bowel Dis. 2011;17:1987–99.
23. Dohan A, Taylor S, Hoeffel C, et al. Diffusion-weighted MRI in Crohn's disease: current status and recommendations. J Magn Reson Imaging. 2016;44:1381–96.
24. Bruining DH, Bhatnagar G, Rimola J, Taylor S, Zimmermann EM, Fletcher JG. CT and MR enterography in Crohn's disease: current and future applications. Abdom Imaging. 2015;40:965–74.

25. Rimola J, Panes J, Ordas I. Magnetic resonance enterography in Crohn's disease: optimal use in clinical practice and clinical trials. Scand J Gastroenterol. 2015;50:66–73.
26. Kumar S, Hakim A, Alexakis C, et al. Small intestinal contrast ultrasonography for the detection of small bowel complications in Crohn's disease: correlation with intraoperative findings and magnetic resonance enterography. J Gastroenterol Hepatol. 2015;30:86–91.
27. Grand DJ, Guglielmo FF, Al-Hawary MM. MR enterography in Crohn's disease: current consensus on optimal imaging technique and future advances from the SAR Crohn's disease-focused panel. Abdom Imaging. 2015;40:953–64.
28. Park SH. DWI at MR Enterography for evaluating bowel inflammation in Crohn disease. AJR Am J Roentgenol. 2016;207:40–8.
29. Rimola J, Alvarez-Cofino A, Perez-Jeldres T, et al. Increasing efficiency of MRE for diagnosis of Crohn's disease activity through proper sequence selection: a practical approach for clinical trials. Abdom Radiol (NY). 2017;42:2783–91.
30. Bhatnagar G, Von Stempel C, Halligan S, Taylor SA. Utility of MR enterography and ultrasound for the investigation of small bowel Crohn's disease. J Magn Reson Imaging. 2017;45:1573–88.
31. Steward MJ, Punwani S, Proctor I, et al. Non-perforating small bowel Crohn's disease assessed by MRI enterography: derivation and histopathological validation of an MR-based activity index. Eur J Radiol. 2012;81:2080–8.
32. Makanyanga JC, Pendse D, Dikaios N, et al. Evaluation of Crohn's disease activity: initial validation of a magnetic resonance enterography global score (MEGS) against faecal calprotectin. Eur Radiol. 2014;24:277–87.
33. Rimola J, Rodriguez S, Garcia-Bosch O, et al. Magnetic resonance for assessment of disease activity and severity in ileocolonic Crohn's disease. Gut. 2009;58:1113–20.
34. Rimola J, Ordas I, Rodriguez S, et al. Magnetic resonance imaging for evaluation of Crohn's disease: validation of parameters of severity and quantitative index of activity. Inflamm Bowel Dis. 2011;17:1759–68.
35. Le Bihan D, Breton E, Lallemand D, Grenier P, Cabanis E, Laval-Jeantet M. MR imaging of intravoxel incoherent motions: application to diffusion and perfusion in neurologic disorders. Radiology. 1986;161:401–7.
36. Chilla GS, Tan CH, Xu C, Poh CL. Diffusion weighted magnetic resonance imaging and its recent trend-a survey. Quant Imaging Med Surg. 2015;5:407–22.
37. Qayyum A. Diffusion-weighted imaging in the abdomen and pelvis: concepts and applications. Radiographics. 2009;29:1797–810.
38. Barral M, Taouli B, Guiu B, et al. Diffusion-weighted MR imaging of the pancreas: current status and recommendations. Radiology. 2015;274:45–63.
39. Tielbeek JA, Ziech ML, Li Z, et al. Evaluation of conventional, dynamic contrast enhanced and diffusion weighted MRI for quantitative Crohn's disease assessment with histopathology of surgical specimens. Eur Radiol. 2014;24:619–29.
40. Hordonneau C, Buisson A, Scanzi J, et al. Diffusion-weighted magnetic resonance imaging in ileocolonic Crohn's disease: validation of quantitative index of activity. Am J Gastroenterol. 2014;109:89–98.
41. Oto A, Kayhan A, Williams JT, et al. Active Crohn's disease in the small bowel: evaluation by diffusion weighted imaging and quantitative dynamic contrast enhanced MR imaging. J Magn Reson Imaging. 2011;33:615–24.
42. Kiryu S, Dodanuki K, Takao H, et al. Free-breathing diffusion-weighted imaging for the assessment of inflammatory activity in Crohn's disease. J Magn Reson Imaging. 2009;29:880–6.
43. Freiman M, Perez-Rossello JM, Callahan MJ, et al. Characterization of fast and slow diffusion from diffusion-weighted MRI of pediatric Crohn's disease. J Magn Reson Imaging. 2013;37:156–63.
44. Neubauer H, Pabst T, Dick A, et al. Small-bowel MRI in children and young adults with Crohn disease: retrospective head-to-head comparison of contrast-enhanced and diffusion-weighted MRI. Pediatr Radiol. 2013;43:103–14.

45. Buisson A, Joubert A, Montoriol PF, et al. Diffusion-weighted magnetic resonance imaging for detecting and assessing ileal inflammation in Crohn's disease. Aliment Pharmacol Ther. 2013;37:537–45.
46. Oussalah A, Laurent V, Bruot O, et al. Diffusion-weighted magnetic resonance without bowel preparation for detecting colonic inflammation in inflammatory bowel disease. Gut. 2010;59:1056–65.
47. Feng Q, Yan YQ, Zhu J, Tong JL, Xu JR. Optimal b value of diffusion-weighted imaging on a 3.0T magnetic resonance scanner in Crohn's disease. World J Gastroenterol. 2014;20:12621–7.
48. Grand DJ, Beland MD, Machan JT, Mayo-Smith WW. Detection of Crohn's disease: comparison of CT and MR enterography without anti-peristaltic agents performed on the same day. Eur J Radiol. 2012;81:1735–41.
49. Grand DJ, Kampalath V, Harris A, et al. MR enterography correlates highly with colonoscopy and histology for both distal ileal and colonic Crohn's disease in 310 patients. Eur J Radiol. 2012;81:e763–9.
50. Park SH, Huh J, Park SH, Lee SS, Kim AY, Yang SK. Diffusion-weighted MR enterography for evaluating Crohn's disease: effect of anti-peristaltic agent on the diagnosis of bowel inflammation. Eur Radiol. 2017;27:2554–62.
51. Stanescu-Siegmund N, Nimsch Y, Wunderlich AP, et al. Quantification of inflammatory activity in patients with Crohn's disease using diffusion weighted imaging (DWI) in MR enteroclysis and MR enterography. Acta Radiol. 2017;58:264–71.
52. Jesuratnam-Nielsen K, Logager VB, Rezanavaz-Gheshlagh B, Munkholm P, Thomsen HS. Plain magnetic resonance imaging as an alternative in evaluating inflammation and bowel damage in inflammatory bowel disease—a prospective comparison with conventional magnetic resonance follow-through. Scand J Gastroenterol. 2015;50:519–27.
53. Cronin CG, Lohan DG, Mhuircheartaigh JN, et al. MRI small-bowel follow-through: prone versus supine patient positioning for best small-bowel distention and lesion detection. AJR Am J Roentgenol. 2008;191:502–6.
54. Caruso A, D'Inca R, Scarpa M, et al. Diffusion-weighted magnetic resonance for assessing ileal Crohn's disease activity. Inflamm Bowel Dis. 2014;20:1575–83.
55. Kim KJ, Lee Y, Park SH, et al. Diffusion-weighted MR enterography for evaluating Crohn's disease: how does it add diagnostically to conventional MR enterography? Inflamm Bowel Dis. 2015;21:101–9.
56. Qi F, Jun S, Qi QY, et al. Utility of the diffusion-weighted imaging for activity evaluation in Crohn's disease patients underwent magnetic resonance enterography. BMC Gastroenterol. 2015;15:12.
57. Foti PV, Farina R, Coronella M, et al. Crohn's disease of the small bowel: evaluation of ileal inflammation by diffusion-weighted MR imaging and correlation with the Harvey-Bradshaw index. Radiol Med. 2015;120:585–94.
58. Li XH, Sun CH, Mao R, et al. Assessment of activity of Crohn disease by diffusion-weighted magnetic resonance imaging. Medicine (Baltimore). 2015;94:e1819.
59. Sato H, Tamura C, Narimatsu K, et al. Magnetic resonance enterocolonography in detecting erosion and redness in intestinal mucosa of patients with Crohn's disease. J Gastroenterol Hepatol. 2015;30:667–73.
60. Church PC, Greer MC, Cytter-Kuint R, et al. Magnetic resonance enterography has good inter-rater agreement and diagnostic accuracy for detecting inflammation in pediatric Crohn disease. Pediatr Radiol. 2017;47:565–75.
61. Oto A, Zhu F, Kulkarni K, Karczmar GS, Turner JR, Rubin D. Evaluation of diffusion-weighted MR imaging for detection of bowel inflammation in patients with Crohn's disease. Acad Radiol. 2009;16:597–603.
62. Seo N, Park SH, Kim KJ, et al. MR Enterography for the evaluation of small-bowel inflammation in Crohn disease by using diffusion-weighted imaging without intravenous contrast material: a prospective noninferiority study. Radiology. 2016;278:762–72.

63. Choi SH, Kim KW, Lee JY, Kim KJ, Park SH. Diffusion-weighted magnetic resonance enterography for evaluating bowel inflammation in Crohn's disease: a systematic review and meta-analysis. Inflamm Bowel Dis. 2016;22:669–79.
64. Plumb AA, Pendse DA, McCartney S, Punwani S, Halligan S, Taylor SA. Lymphoid nodular hyperplasia of the terminal ileum can mimic active crohn disease on MR enterography. AJR Am J Roentgenol. 2014;203:W400–7.
65. Daperno M, D'Haens G, Van Assche G, et al. Development and validation of a new, simplified endoscopic activity score for Crohn's disease: the SES-CD. Gastrointest Endosc. 2004;60:505–12.
66. Ream JM, Dillman JR, Adler J, et al. MRI diffusion-weighted imaging (DWI) in pediatric small bowel Crohn disease: correlation with MRI findings of active bowel wall inflammation. Pediatr Radiol. 2013;43:1077–85.
67. Buisson A, Hordonneau C, Goutte M, Boyer L, Pereira B, Bommelaer G. Diffusion-weighted magnetic resonance imaging is effective to detect ileocolonic ulcerations in Crohn's disease. Aliment Pharmacol Ther. 2015;42:452–60.
68. Bhatnagar G, Dikaios N, Prezzi D, Vega R, Halligan S, Taylor SA. Changes in dynamic contrast-enhanced pharmacokinetic and diffusion-weighted imaging parameters reflect response to anti-TNF therapy in Crohn's disease. Br J Radiol. 2015;88:20150547.
69. Huh J, Kim KJ, Park SH, et al. Diffusion-weighted MR Enterography to monitor bowel inflammation after medical therapy in Crohn's disease: a prospective longitudinal study. Korean J Radiol. 2017;18:162–72.
70. Dillman JR, Smith EA, Sanchez R, et al. DWI in pediatric small-bowel Crohn disease: are apparent diffusion coefficients surrogates for disease activity in patients receiving infliximab therapy? AJR Am J Roentgenol. 2016;207:1002–8.
71. Kanda T, Fukusato T, Matsuda M, et al. Gadolinium-based contrast agent accumulates in the brain even in subjects without severe renal dysfunction: evaluation of autopsy brain specimens with inductively coupled plasma mass spectroscopy. Radiology. 2015;276:228–32.
72. Dubron C, Avni F, Boutry N, Turck D, Duhamel A, Amzallag-Bellenger E. Prospective evaluation of free-breathing diffusion-weighted imaging for the detection of inflammatory bowel disease with MR enterography in childhood population. Br J Radiol. 2016;89:20150840.
73. Alkim C, Alkim H, Koksal AR, Boga S, Sen I. Angiogenesis in inflammatory bowel disease. Int J Inflam. 2015;2015:970890.
74. Bacaner MB. Quantitative measurement of regional colon blood flow in the normal and pathological human bowel. Gastroenterology. 1966;51:764–77.
75. Rutella S, Fiorino G, Vetrano S, et al. Infliximab therapy inhibits inflammation-induced angiogenesis in the mucosa of patients with Crohn's disease. Am J Gastroenterol. 2011;106:762–70.
76. Padhani AR. Dynamic contrast-enhanced MRI in clinical oncology: current status and future directions. J Magn Reson Imaging. 2002;16:407–22.
77. Oommen J, Oto A. Contrast-enhanced MRI of the small bowel in Crohn's disease. Abdom Imaging. 2011;36:134–41.
78. Boijsen E, Ekman CA, Lundh G. Selective splanchnic angiography. Adv Surg. 1968;3:13–73.
79. Pendse DA, Makanyanga JC, Plumb AA, et al. Diffusion-weighted imaging for evaluating inflammatory activity in Crohn's disease: comparison with histopathology, conventional MRI activity scores, and faecal calprotectin. Abdom Radiol (NY). 2017;42:115–23.
80. Choi D, Jin Lee S, Ah Cho Y, et al. Bowel wall thickening in patients with Crohn's disease: CT patterns and correlation with inflammatory activity. Clin Radiol. 2003;58:68–74.
81. Tolan DJ, Greenhalgh R, Zealley IA, Halligan S, Taylor SA. MR enterographic manifestations of small bowel Crohn disease. Radiographics. 2010;30:367–84.
82. Roccarina D, Garcovich M, Ainora ME, et al. Diagnosis of bowel diseases: the role of imaging and ultrasonography. World J Gastroenterol. 2013;19:2144–53.
83. Alkim C, Savas B, Ensari A, et al. Expression of p53, VEGF, microvessel density, and cyclin-D1 in noncancerous tissue of inflammatory bowel disease. Dig Dis Sci. 2009;54:1979–84.
84. Danese S, Fiorino G, Angelucci E, et al. Narrow-band imaging endoscopy to assess mucosal angiogenesis in inflammatory bowel disease: a pilot study. World J Gastroenterol. 2010;16:2396–400.

85. Taylor SA, Punwani S, Rodriguez-Justo M, et al. Mural Crohn disease: correlation of dynamic contrast-enhanced MR imaging findings with angiogenesis and inflammation at histologic examination—pilot study. Radiology. 2009;251:369–79.
86. Makanyanga J, Punwani S, Taylor SA. Assessment of wall inflammation and fibrosis in Crohn's disease: value of T1-weighted gadolinium-enhanced MR imaging. Abdom Imaging. 2012;37:933–43.
87. Li Z, Tielbeek JAW, Caan MWA, et al. Expiration-phase template-based motion correction of free-breathing abdominal dynamic contrast enhanced MRI. IEEE Trans Biomed Eng. 2015;62:1215–25.
88. Melbourne A, Atkinson D, White MJ, Collins D, Leach M, Hawkes D. Registration of dynamic contrast-enhanced MRI using a progressive principal component registration (PPCR). Phys Med Biol. 2007;52:5147–56.
89. Hamy V, Dikaios N, Punwani S, et al. Respiratory motion correction in dynamic MRI using robust data decomposition registration—application to DCE-MRI. Med Image Anal. 2014;18:301–13.
90. Tofts PS, Brix G, Buckley DL, et al. Estimating kinetic parameters from dynamic contrast-enhanced T(1)-weighted MRI of a diffusable tracer: standardized quantities and symbols. J Magn Reson Imaging. 1999;10:223–32.
91. Maccioni F, Viscido A, Broglia L, et al. Evaluation of Crohn disease activity with magnetic resonance imaging. Abdom Imaging. 2000;25:219–28.
92. Sempere GA, Martinez Sanjuan V, Medina Chulia E, et al. MRI evaluation of inflammatory activity in Crohn's disease. AJR Am J Roentgenol. 2005;184:1829–35.
93. Pupillo VA, Di Cesare E, Frieri G, Limbucci N, Tanga M, Masciocchi C. Assessment of inflammatory activity in Crohn's disease by means of dynamic contrast-enhanced MRI. Radiol Med. 2007;112:798–809.
94. Del Vescovo R, Sansoni I, Caviglia R, et al. Dynamic contrast enhanced magnetic resonance imaging of the terminal ileum: differentiation of activity of Crohn's disease. Abdom Imaging. 2008;33:417–24.
95. Knuesel PR, Kubik RA, Crook DW, Eigenmann F, Froehlich JM. Assessment of dynamic contrast enhancement of the small bowel in active Crohn's disease using 3D MR enterography. Eur J Radiol. 2010;73:607–13.
96. Oto A, Fan X, Mustafi D, et al. Quantitative analysis of dynamic contrast enhanced MRI for assessment of bowel inflammation in Crohn's disease pilot study. Acad Radiol. 2009;16:1223–30.
97. Horsthuis K, Nederveen AJ, de Feiter MW, Lavini C, Stokkers PC, Stoker J. Mapping of T1-values and gadolinium-concentrations in MRI as indicator of disease activity in luminal Crohn's disease: a feasibility study. J Magn Reson Imaging. 2009;29:488–93.
98. Giusti S, Faggioni L, Neri E, et al. Dynamic MRI of the small bowel: usefulness of quantitative contrast-enhancement parameters and time-signal intensity curves for differentiating between active and inactive Crohn's disease. Abdom Imaging. 2010;35:646–53.
99. Rottgen R, Grandke T, Grieser C, Lehmkuhl L, Hamm B, Ludemann L. Measurement of MRI enhancement kinetics for evaluation of inflammatory activity in Crohn's disease. Clin Imaging. 2010;34:29–35.
100. Florie J, Wasser MN, Arts-Cieslik K, Akkerman EM, Siersema PD, Stoker J. Dynamic contrast-enhanced MRI of the bowel wall for assessment of disease activity in Crohn's disease. AJR Am J Roentgenol. 2006;186:1384–92.
101. Ziech ML, Lavini C, Caan MW, et al. Dynamic contrast-enhanced MRI in patients with luminal Crohn's disease. Eur J Radiol. 2012;81:3019–27.
102. van Schie JJN, Lavini C, van Vliet LJ, et al. Estimating the arterial input function from dynamic contrast-enhanced MRI data with compensation for flow enhancement (II): applications in spine diagnostics and assessment of Crohn's disease. J Magn Reson Imaging. 2017;47(5):1197–204.
103. Zhu J, Zhang F, Zhou J, Li H. Assessment of therapeutic response in Crohn's disease using quantitative dynamic contrast enhanced MRI (DCE-MRI) parameters: a preliminary study. Medicine (Baltimore). 2017;96:e7759.

104. Patel P, Ormanoski M, Hoadley KM. Magnetic resonance enterography findings in Crohn's disease in the pediatric population and correlation with fluoroscopic and multidetector computed tomographic techniques. J Clin Imaging Sci. 2011;1:41.
105. Maccioni F, Patak MA, Signore A, Laghi A. New frontiers of MRI in Crohn's disease: motility imaging, diffusion-weighted imaging, perfusion MRI, MR spectroscopy, molecular imaging, and hybrid imaging (PET/MRI). Abdom Imaging. 2012;37:974–82.
106. de Jonge CS, Gollifer RM, Nederveen AJ, et al. Dynamic MRI for bowel motility imaging-how fast and how long? Br J Radiol. 2018:20170845.
107. de Jonge CS, Smout A, Nederveen AJ, Stoker J. Evaluation of gastrointestinal motility with MRI: advances, challenges and opportunities. Neurogastroenterol Motil 2018;30(1). doi: https://doi.org/10.1111/nmo.13257.
108. Ghobrial PM, Neuberger I, Guglielmo FF, et al. Cine MR enterography grading of small bowel peristalsis: evaluation of the antiperistaltic effectiveness of sublingual hyoscyamine sulfate. Acad Radiol. 2014;21:86–91.
109. Bickelhaupt S, Froehlich JM, Cattin R, et al. Software-assisted quantitative analysis of small bowel motility compared to manual measurements. Clin Radiol. 2014;69:363–71.
110. Odille F, Menys A, Ahmed A, Punwani S, Taylor SA, Atkinson D. Quantitative assessment of small bowel motility by nonrigid registration of dynamic MR images. Magn Reson Med. 2012;68:783–93.
111. Froehlich JM, Waldherr C, Stoupis C, Erturk SM, Patak MA. MR motility imaging in Crohn's disease improves lesion detection compared with standard MR imaging. Eur Radiol. 2010;20:1945–51.
112. Menys A, Atkinson D, Odille F, et al. Quantified terminal ileal motility during MR enterography as a potential biomarker of Crohn's disease activity: a preliminary study. Eur Radiol. 2012;22:2494–501.
113. Cullmann JL, Bickelhaupt S, Froehlich JM, et al. MR imaging in Crohn's disease: correlation of MR motility measurement with histopathology in the terminal ileum. Neurogastroenterol Motil. 2013;25:749-e577.
114. Hahnemann ML, Nensa F, Kinner S, et al. Quantitative assessment of small bowel motility in patients with Crohn's disease using dynamic MRI. Neurogastroenterol Motil. 2015;27:841–8.
115. Akerman A, Mansson S, Fork FT, et al. Computational postprocessing quantification of small bowel motility using magnetic resonance images in clinical practice: an initial experience. J Magn Reson Imaging. 2016;44:277–87.
116. Plumb AA, Menys A, Russo E, et al. Magnetic resonance imaging-quantified small bowel motility is a sensitive marker of response to medical therapy in Crohn's disease. Aliment Pharmacol Ther. 2015;42:343–55.
117. Menys A, Makanyanga J, Plumb A, et al. Aberrant motility in unaffected small bowel is linked to inflammatory burden and patient symptoms in Crohn's disease. Inflamm Bowel Dis. 2016;22:424–32.
118. Bickelhaupt S, Pazahr S, Chuck N, et al. Crohn's disease: small bowel motility impairment correlates with inflammatory-related markers C-reactive protein and calprotectin. Neurogastroenterol Motil. 2013;25:467–73.
119. Sotoudeh H, Sharma A, Fowler KJ, McConathy J, Dehdashti F. Clinical application of PET/MRI in oncology. J Magn Reson Imaging. 2016;44:265–76.
120. Malide D, Davies-Hill TM, Levine M, Simpson IA. Distinct localization of GLUT-1, -3, and -5 in human monocyte-derived macrophages: effects of cell activation. Am J Phys. 1998;274:E516–26.
121. Neurath MF, Vehling D, Schunk K, et al. Noninvasive assessment of Crohn's disease activity: a comparison of 18F-fluorodeoxyglucose positron emission tomography, hydromagnetic resonance imaging, and granulocyte scintigraphy with labeled antibodies. Am J Gastroenterol. 2002;97:1978–85.
122. Louis E, Ancion G, Colard A, Spote V, Belaiche J, Hustinx R. Noninvasive assessment of Crohn's disease intestinal lesions with (18)F-FDG PET/CT. J Nucl Med. 2007;48:1053–9.

123. Bettenworth D, Reuter S, Hermann S, et al. Translational 18F-FDG PET/CT imaging to monitor lesion activity in intestinal inflammation. J Nucl Med. 2013;54:748–55.
124. Groshar D, Bernstine H, Stern D, et al. PET/CT enterography in Crohn disease: correlation of disease activity on CT enterography with 18F-FDG uptake. J Nucl Med. 2010;51:1009–14.
125. Saboury B, Salavati A, Brothers A, et al. FDG PET/CT in Crohn's disease: correlation of quantitative FDG PET/CT parameters with clinical and endoscopic surrogate markers of disease activity. Eur J Nucl Med Mol Imaging. 2014;41:605–14.
126. Russo EA, Khan S, Janisch R, et al. Role of 18F-fluorodeoxyglucose positron emission tomography in the monitoring of inflammatory activity in Crohn's disease. Inflamm Bowel Dis. 2016;22:2619–29.
127. Jadvar H, Colletti PM. Competitive advantage of PET/MRI. Eur J Radiol. 2014;83:84–94.
128. Pellino G, Nicolai E, Catalano OA, et al. PET/MR versus PET/CT imaging: impact on the clinical management of small-bowel Crohn's disease. J Crohns Colitis. 2016;10:277–85.
129. Catalano OA, Gee MS, Nicolai E, et al. Evaluation of quantitative PET/MR enterography biomarkers for discrimination of inflammatory strictures from fibrotic strictures in Crohn disease. Radiology. 2016;278:792–800.
130. Rieder F, Zimmermann EM, Remzi FH, Sandborn WJ. Crohn's disease complicated by strictures: a systematic review. Gut. 2013;62:1072–84.
131. Lenze F, Wessling J, Bremer J, et al. Detection and differentiation of inflammatory versus fibromatous Crohn's disease strictures: prospective comparison of 18F-FDG-PET/CT, MR-enteroclysis, and transabdominal ultrasound versus endoscopic/histologic evaluation. Inflamm Bowel Dis. 2012;18:2252–60.

Role of Imaging in Detecting Bowel Fibrosis and Bowel Damage

7

Cristiana Bonifacio, Nicolò Gennaro, and Gionata Fiorino

Abstract

Imaging plays a key role in the comprehensive assessment of bowel structural damage. Radiology is fundamental to confirm the initial diagnosis and the extent of disease along the digestive tract. Moreover, imaging is a critical tool in the monitoring of the response to drug therapy. In this chapter, technique, indications and limitations of the major imaging methods used in the assessment of CD (ultrasound, computed tomography, magnetic resonance imaging) are reviewed. A special focus is dedicated to the detection and quantification of bowel fibrosis and bowel wall damage with CT and MRI. Future perspectives are finally reviewed according to the latest developments in imaging technology.

C. Bonifacio (✉)
Department of Radiology, Humanitas Research Hospital, Via Alessandro Manzoni 56, Milan, Italy
e-mail: cristiana.bonifacio@humanitas.it

N. Gennaro
Department of Radiology, Humanitas Research Hospital, Humanitas University, Training School in Radiology, Via Rita Levi Montalcini 4, Milan, Italy

G. Fiorino
IBD Center, Department of Gastroenterology, Humanitas Research Hospital, Via Alessandro Manzoni 56, Milan, Italy

Department of Biomedical Sciences, Humanitas University, Via Alessandro Manzoni 56, Milan, Italy

J. Rimola (ed.), *Cross-Sectional Imaging in Crohn's Disease*,
https://doi.org/10.1007/978-3-319-96586-4_7

7.1 Introduction

Crohn's disease (CD) is a destructive, progressive, and disabling inflammatory bowel disease (IBD), potentially involving the gastrointestinal tract from the mouth to anus. Some segments are more involved than others, like ileum and the proximal colonic tract [1]. It is a lifelong condition, progressive but with a typical intermittent activity, characterized by prolonged remission intervals and sudden aggressive recurrences. Despite a purely inflammatory onset of the disease, over 30% of patients develop bowel fibrogenesis (11–44% already at the time of diagnosis) [2], due to the poorly controlled healing process triggered by chronic transmural inflammation. The exact biological mechanisms of fibrosis deposition are still under investigation, but latest evidences confirmed the synergic role of TGF-beta, VEGF, PDGF-alpha, PKC, RAS, RAF, and ERK proteins drawing a complex interplay of genetic, microbial, and immunological factors. Abnormal deposition of extracellular matrix (ECM) is the end product of these molecular cascades, resulting in strictures, scar formation, and tissue distortion. Unfortunately, since bowel fibrosis is irreversible and not responsive to available medications, it usually requires surgical resection with a cumulative anatomical and structural damage. Like fibrotic strictures, fistulae are also common complication of the chronic inflammatory pattern of CD resulting in a permanent bowel damage that usually requires surgery which removes complications but causes further structural damage [3]. Disease eventually recurs in 17–55% of patients at 5 years and 72–73% of patients at 20 years after surgery, leading to new surgical resections in up to 11–32% of cases at 5 years and 46–55% of cases at 20 years [4], with consequent increase in the cumulative bowel damage, loss of quality of life, and disability [5].

The CD phenotypes are classified as non-stricturing non-penetrating [B1], stricturing [B2], and penetrating disease [B3], according to the Montreal classification [6]. Longitudinal follow-up studies have shown that only 40% of patients classified in the B1 group won't evolve in the stricturing or penetrating group [7, 8]. Prevention of organ damage through an early effective therapy represents a crucial endpoint beyond long-term clinical remission that can impact on the long-term evolution of the disease [9, 10].

7.2 Structural Damage

Imaging plays a key role in the comprehensive assessment of bowel structural damage. Firstly, it is fundamental to confirm the initial diagnosis (f.e. to distinguish Crohn's disease from ulcerous colitis) and the extent of disease along the digestive tract. Secondly, cross-sectional imaging techniques allow to assess and track the progression of extraintestinal CD manifestations. Moreover, imaging assesses disease activity in CD patients with symptomatic recurrence and represents an important tool in the monitoring of the response to drug therapy. Given its chronic nature, CD needs careful lifelong monitoring to successfully prevent complications and offer the best treatment for the patient. Imaging plays a major role in this continuous assessment, providing an accurate anatomic description of the location and length of CD lesions along the digestive tract, and recently also functional features of the disease have been collected, thanks to the achievement of functional MRI sequences. With many drug therapies for CD being investigated and introduced in the clinical practice, imaging has established as a tool to monitor the response to CD therapy and the progression of bowel damage [11–13]. Routine medical imaging for CD includes high-resolution ultrasound, CT-enterography, and MRI-enterography. Endoscopy is also a valuable technique to describe the bowel mucosa but provides just the mucosal assessment with a limited access to the small bowel. Similarly, video-capsule endoscopy does visualize the entire small bowel but cannot provide tissue sampling, and it is contraindicated in obstructed patients. All these intrinsic limitations of the endoscopic assessment make transmural examinations like CT and MRI the two fundamental imaging techniques to yield a rigorous and comprehensive assessment of CD.

Bowel damage in Crohn's disease (CD) is referred as a spectrum of heterogeneous lesions involving all intestinal layers, ranging from irreversible fibrotic strictures causing luminal narrowing with prestenotic dilatation to abscess, fistulas, aphthous, and deep ulcers [14, 15]. Moreover, active inflammation can coexist with irreversible fibrotic or penetrating lesion [16, 17]. Taking into consideration the Montreal classification, bowel damage is defined as the progression from B1 to B2 and B3, which occurs in the 30–60% of cases in the long term [18]. Bowel damage can be also defined as the presence of strictures, fistulas, or abscesses [14]. Measuring cumulative bowel damage is critical to understand the progression of the disease and to draw an effective treatment plan to prevent it. CD typically starts with a non-stricturing non-penetrating pattern (B1) and evolves to stricturing and/or penetrating during the disease course (B2–B3) [8]. However, stricturing or penetrating complications are present in up to 20–50% at onset, suggesting that early diagnosis and early treatment may be crucial to prevent from structural damage and disease progression. Moreover, as stated by Fiorino et al. [14], the presence of CD-related complications detected by cross-sectional imaging at diagnosis is associated with higher risk of surgery and hospitalizations compared to those without complications. Cross-sectional imaging techniques are the best modalities to depict bowel damage. In particular, US and MRI seem to have the best reproducibility and high sensitivity and specificity in detecting intestinal and extraintestinal damage especially in proximal small bowel, without the risk related to ionizing radiations [19]. On the other hand, if MRI and CT can confidently describe extra-luminal complications like abscesses, fistulas, or the perianal disease [20, 21], endoscopy is complementary to imaging in the detection and evaluation of intraluminal complications, like fibrotic intestinal strictures [22, 23]. The International Program to develop New Indexes in Crohn's disease (IPNIC) group has worked in the last decade on the integration of MRI findings with endoscopy and clinical history of previous surgery. These efforts lead to the development of the active measure of CD bowel damage, the Lémann index [24], a classification index-based endoscopy, imaging findings (CT and MRI), and surgical history. The Lémann index takes into account strictures, penetration by ulcers, fistulas, abscess, and surgical resection of bowel in each segment for the four CD locations (upper digestive tract, small bowel, colon/rectum, perianal/anal). One major advantage of the Lémann score with regard to other classification systems (e.g., the Montreal classification) is the possibility to quantify the severity of the structural bowel damage. This is particularly useful when measuring bowel damage progression with repeated assessments over time.

7.3 MRI Technique and Assessment of Bowel Damage

Bowel damage is the result of both active and chronic phases of the disease. The active phase is characterized by exacerbation of clinical symptoms laboratory and markers indicative of active inflammation. When assessing bowel damage, MRI plays the fundamental role. 1.5 T or 3 T MR enterography provides both morphological and functional information through conventional MR sequences and dynamic contrast-enhanced (DCE) MRI with diffusion-weighted imaging (DWI). An MRE-based score (MR index) has been developed that has proven to be useful in measuring the activity and severity of CD, alongside the currently used validated endoscopic scores [25]. The MR index has a high accuracy for the detection of disease activity and the detection of ulcerative lesions (Fig. 7.1).

In the acute inflammatory state, MRI shows wall thickening >3 mm (due to acute inflammation or fibrosis), ulcerations, fistulas, and mural and peripheral edema all characterized by hyperintensity in T2-W fat-suppressed/fluid-sensitive sequences, surrounded by a halo of T2-W intermediate signal (Fig. 7.2).

The acute edematous wall can cause stricturing even in the acute phase of the disease, mimicking a chronic fibrostenotic stricture.

Common findings of chronic CD are the fibro-fatty changes of the mesentery, fibrotic strictures, and fistulas, which are better displayed with fast spin echo or contrast-enhanced T1-W sequences. The degree of inflammation correlates well with the hyperintensity on T2-W due to edema, the presence of ulcerations, and blurred margins. By acquiring contrast-enhanced CT or MRI, an early submucosal and serosal hyperenhancement together with the edematous submucosa make the bowel wall appear thickened and markedly layered, with a target appearance. These characteristics of active inflammation are positive predictors of response to anti-TNF agents. Moreover, a significant association exists between T2 hyperintensity, ulceration, inner wall hyperenhancement, blurred margin, wall thickness, and degree of histological inflammation. Since CD is a transmural pathology, a diffuse enhancement may be seen extending toward the mesentery during the active phase. Finally, deep ulcers appear as a high-signal T2-W serpiginous images that alternate with thickened mucosal folds (the so-called cobblestone appearance) [26, 27].

Parameters like the presence of edema, ulcers, pseudopolyps, lymph node enlargement, mural thickness, T1-W bowel wall ratio, T2-W bowel wall ratio, DCE MRI maximum enhancement (ME), initial slope of increase (ISI), time to peak (TTP), and apparent diffusion coefficient (ADC) on DWI allow for a comprehensive evaluation of CD-related damage [27]. A moderate and significant correlation was found among mural thickness, T1 ratio, T2 mural/CSF ratio, ME, ISI, and

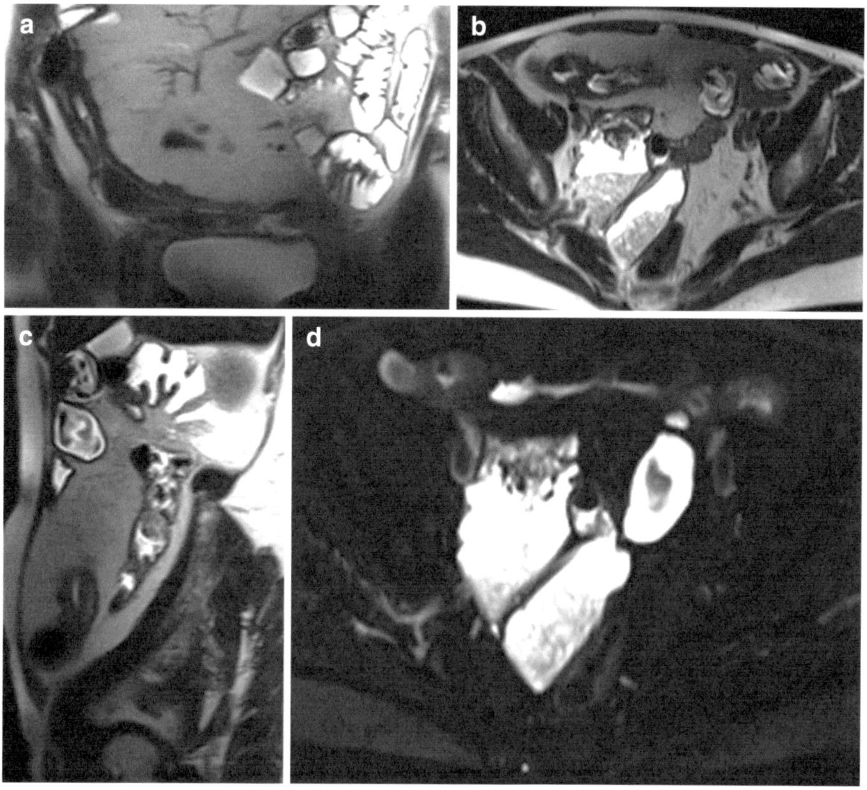

Fig. 7.1 (**a**) Coronal, (**b**) axial, and (**c**) sagittal planes in a T2-W sequence showing a distal ileum involvement of CD with stenosis, wall thickening, submucosal edema, and perivisceral fat stranding. (**d**) T2-W FS shows submucosal edema. MRI findings are consistent with active inflammation

inflammation [27]. Moreover, mural thickness, T1 ratio, T2 mural/CSF ratio, ME, ISI, and ADC values also showed significant differences between grades of fibro-stenosis. T2 mural/CSF ratio can be used to discriminate between inflammation and fibrosis. Interestingly, mural thickness and T1 ratio correlated with both AIS and FS in the study by Tielbeek et al. [27]. These findings support the hypothesis that inflammation and fibrosis are not excluding processes [28]), even in the same bowel segment [29, 30]. Also DCE MRI correlated well with the histopathological specimens in assessing CD activity, since ME and ISI correlated well with a histopathology-based reference standard. DCE MRI confirms to be of additional value to the conventional MRI protocol in order to facilitate better grading of Crohn's disease activity.

Finally, accurate detection and grading of bowel fibrosis are pivotal to optimize patient's selection for potential responsiveness to antifibrotic agents that are now under clinical validation [31–33]. CT and MRI gave similar results for the detection of bowel wall thickening >3 mm. MRI easily detects signs of bowel wall edema in

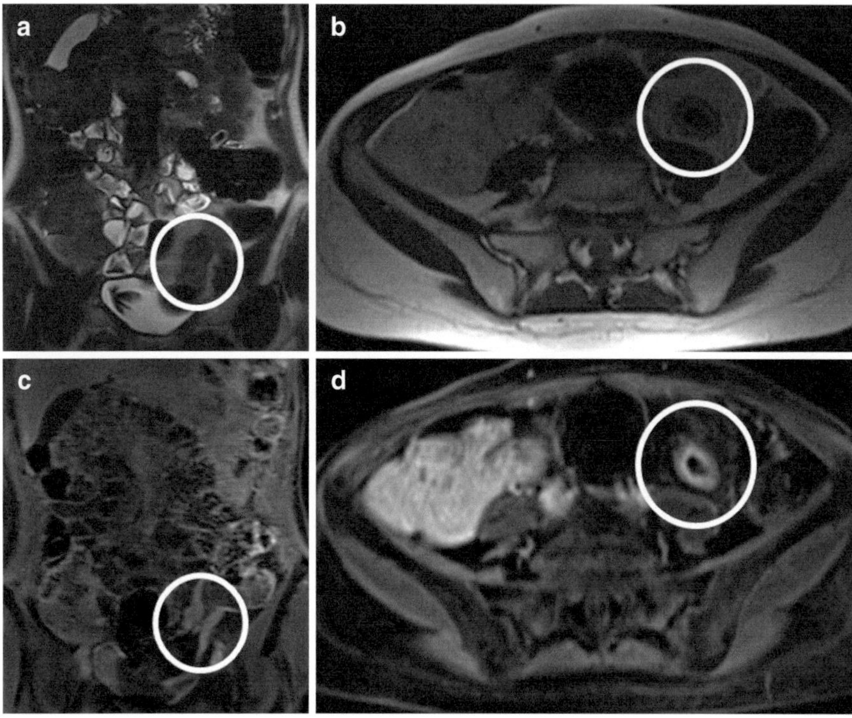

Fig. 7.2 T2-W sequence in coronal (**a**) and axial (**b**) view shows sigmoid involvement of CD with stenosis and wall thickening. T1-W after Gd administration shows extensive wall enhancement, in coronal (**c**) and axial plane (**d**)

T2W and has been shown to be as sensitive as CT in the evaluation of extraintestinal abdominal signs of CD, such as involvement of perivisceral fat and abdominal adenopathies. In the evaluation of enteroenteric fistulas, CT accuracy is similar to MRI, although for both techniques sensitivity, specificity, and accuracy have been described as less than 50%.

Finally, neither CT nor MR is sufficiently sensitive and specific for the detection of purely mucosal lesions, and there is still not enough evidence supporting their alternative role to endoscopy in assessing mucosal healing.

7.3.1 Technical Notes for MRI in CD

MRI, with a 91% of specificity and sensitivity, can be considered as the reference imaging technology for assessment of CD. Two techniques are traditionally available: MRI-enterography and MRI-enteroclysis. The latter consists in the administration of oral contrast through a nasojejunal tube but has been replaced by the more common MRI-enterography.

MRI-enterography is the most common MRI technique and is performed after the ingestion for 1–2 L of hyperosmolar oral contrast solution, like 2.5% mannitol solution, barium sulfate, or polyethylene glycol (PEG), with the patient fasting for at least 6 h. The oral contrast medium appears typically low on T1-W and high in signal on T2-W. Glucagon can be used as a spasmolytic drug, and a rectal enema may be useful to increase the visualization of the terminal ileum. Study protocol includes the acquisition of coronal and axial images using a phased array coil and a high-field (1.5–3.0 T) magnet. True fast imaging with steady-state precession and HASTE sequences with and without fat suppression are usually obtained. Fast-suppressed coronal and axial (or three-dimensional) T1-W breath-hold/VIBE gradient echo of the abdomen and pelvis are finally required, before and 70s and 7 minutes after intravenous contrast administration, to evaluate the presence of fibrosis. Moreover, DWI assessment has been increasingly inserted in the CD MRI protocol. Being the DWI inversely related to the cell density, an acutely inflamed area will appear as an area of restricted diffusion (hyperintense) with decreased ADC values. Despite the discomfort of a large amount of liquid, the high costs of the examination, the difficulty to hold the breath intermittently, and the long MR acquisition times, MRI provides excellent details of ulcers, mural penetration, wall thickening, hyperemia, and peri-intestinal reactive structures without exposing the patients to the risks of ionizing radiations.

7.4 Detection of Fibrosis

Fibrosis is the result of a chronic inflammation and is a cause of major complications like bowel obstruction. Among the many classifications proposed to quantify fibrosis in CD, the Montreal classification [17] is the most common. CD patients that develop fibrosis are labeled as Montreal class B2 inflammatory phenotype.

Fibrosis deposition occurs predominantly in deep layers of the bowel. Limited edema, a compact tissue, and a reduced number and diameter of the vessels compared with the normal mucosa are typical findings inside the fibrotic areas.

Since treatment options are formulated on the discrimination between active inflammatory and fibrotic-predominant lesions, a major challenge for medical imaging is to differentiate lesions that can still respond to medical treatment (inflammatory-related) from the ones that benefit only from endoscopic balloon dilatation or surgical resection (fibrotic-related bowel thickening) [3, 34, 35]. At this regard, both MRI and CT can detect fibrosis with direct and indirect signs, but MR enteroclysis is significantly more sensitive than CT (with and without contrast administration) to detect intestinal stricture (sensitivity 57% vs 42%, specificity 82% vs 68%). Postoperative recurrence of fibrostenosis has been investigated with CT virtual colonoscopy, but its diagnostic performance has not overpassed colonoscopy yet.

In order to maximize the visibility of the strictures, enterography technique (CT or MRI), better if performed after enteroclysis, is the best choice [36]. Pseudosacculations in the antimesenteric side of the bowel wall indicate presence of fibrosis [37]. Mural thickness, edema, and stratification have been found to correlate with fibrosis, but a global agreement has not been met yet.

The intestinal stenotic tract appears thickened, proportionally to the histological degree of fibrosis, and suffers usually a luminal narrowing. Decrease of signal intensity of the thickened bowel wall or low bowel-wall signal intensity, fat-saturated T2-weighted MRI images, and a reduction in bowel-wall early enhancement or absent or minimal transmural enhancement on gadolinium contrast MR are usually associated with intestinal fibrosis. MRI can therefore potentially distinguish between patients with fibrosis and superimposed inflammation and those with chronic fibrosis [38].

However, signal intensity is not always decreased in T2W within the fibrotic areas. Higher T2 mural/CSF ratios have been significantly associated with more inflammation as well as mild fibrostenosis, whereas low T2 mural/CSF ratio is significantly associated with low inflammation scores and with severe fibrostenosis. Decrease in ADC values also correlated significantly with fibrostenosis [27]. Even if fibrosis is better evaluated with MRI, it still can be detected on CT due to indirect signs like bowel sacculations, dilatations, and mural thickness.

DCE MRI represents an added value in the assessment of the CD activity. Even if an early contrast enhancement is not found in the fibrotic areas, later, contrast-enhanced phase shows a homogenous pattern of enhancement that progresses over time along with the natural history of the disease (Fig. 7.3).

Rimola et al. described different patterns of enhancement at 70s and at 7 min, representing the two phases with the higher predicting value for CD activity [39]. At 70 s, three patterns are known: enhancement of superficial (mucosal) layer, homogeneous enhancement (all bowel wall enhancing equally), and layered enhancement

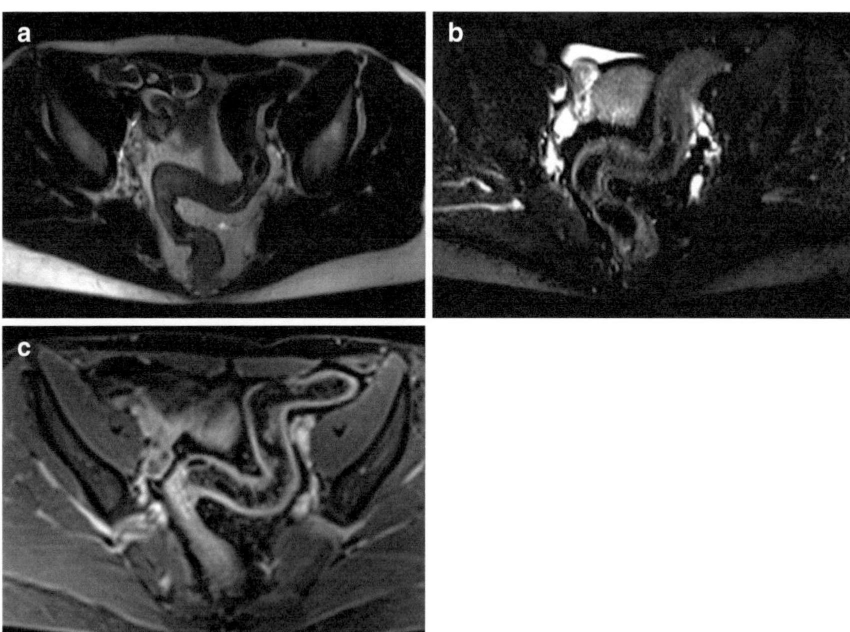

Fig. 7.3 (**a**) T2-W sequence shows rectal and sigmoid wall thickening in patient with CD. (**b**) T2-W FS shows submucosal mild edema. (**c**) T1-W sequence after Gd administration shows mild mucosal enhancement in the late phase. MRI findings suggest fibrotic evolution

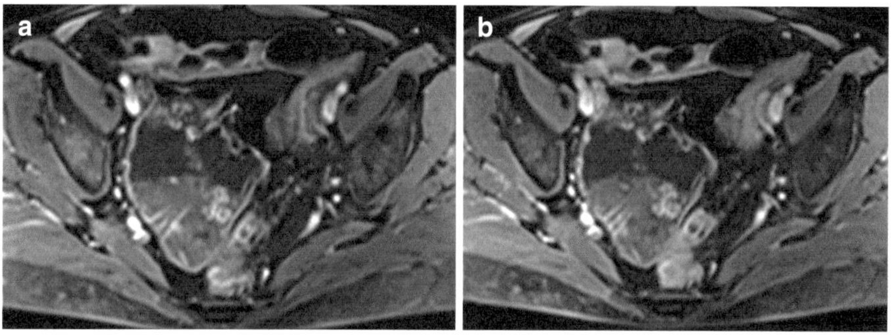

Fig. 7.4 (**a**) T1-W FS after Gd administration shows mucosal enhancement in the venous phase that does not increase in the late phase (**b**). No fibrosis is therefore suspected

(both mucosa-submucosa and serosa enhancing, with an in-between band of poor enhancement). Even if at 70 s the more superficial layers show a slightly increased contrast enhancement, at 7 min, each layer (deep and superficial) shows a similar hyperenhanced appearance. A homogenous pattern of enhancement at 70 s, an increased signal intensity in T2-W, and a progressive contrast enhancement >25% between 70 s and 7 min have been demonstrated to be a possible indicator of fibrosis [39], although these findings need to be validated in further studies (Fig. 7.4).

7.5 Ultrasound

Ultrasound (US) is a routine imaging technique for the assessment of CD patients. Some current applications of US and its implementations like color Doppler and CEUS are monitoring the activity of the disease, especially in pediatric patients or when a good-quality MRI scan may be complicated to achieve. A proper US examination requires a high-frequency probe and a multiplanar image acquisition of the whole abdomen. A pre-FAST scan is recommended, and a full bladder provides an acoustic window for the assessment of the pelvic bowel loops. CEUS can provide information about the microvascular density of the thickened bowel wall since US contrast agents like polyethylene glycol solution do not have the interstitial phase, drawing a direct correlation between vascularization and the contrast enhancement [2, 40–42]. Ultrasound elastography is also showing some potential in evaluating bowel wall fibrosis and in discriminating between active or chronic inflammation. Moreover, wall stiffness measurement seems to be an emerging tool to detect the presence of severe fibrosis in a stenotic intestinal tract [43]. Strain differences in the pathological bowel tracts have been directly associated with increased muscular fibers and collagen deposition and allow to discriminate low-grade from high-grade bowel wall fibrosis in ex vivo human intestinal specimens [44].

Common findings of CD in ultrasound are bowel wall thickening (large bowel wall >3 mm, small bowel wall >2.5 mm), strictures associated with prestenotic dilatation, a decrease of normal peristalsis, duct-like structures representing fistulas, and fibro-fatty, echogenic, and hyperemic changes of the mesentery associated with local lymphadenopathies. A scoring system, the sonographic lesion index for CD (SLIC), has been recently proposed by Calabrese et al., based on the small intestine contrast ultrasonography (SICUS), which unfortunately lacks of good reproducibility due to its complexity, thus limiting its wide adoption [45, 46].

7.6 Computed Tomography

Computed tomography (CT) is a widely available, time-sparing, cross-sectional imaging method that allows diagnosis and monitoring of CD.

In the active phase of the disease, CT provides visualization of mural stratification and thickening, submucosal fat deposition, fat stranding around the bowel wall, and the presence of lymphadenopathies. Since the late 1990s, contrast-enhanced CT has entered in clinical practice for the evaluation of CD. After injection of iodized intravenous contrast medium, wall hyperemia can be quantified, and typical finding of active inflammation like the "comb sign" due to the distended vasa recta of the intestinal arcades in the mesentery can be found. Deep mural ulcers can be better visualized with MRI than with CT. On the contrary, acute emergencies like pneumoperitoneum due to visceral perforation, toxic megacolon with its classic appearance of loss of haustral folds, mural thinning, and dilation >6 cm are optimally displayed by CT intestinal and extraintestinal complications of CD like abscess, perforation, fistula, or bowel obstruction which can easily be described with contrast enhanced CT.

In the chronic phase, fat proliferation can be found in the mesentery as well as submucosal fat deposition in the affected bowel tracts. Despite the good diagnostic performance and the relatively inexpensive costs when compared to MRI, CT still presents the disadvantage of ionizing radiation exposure (reduced from to 15 mSv to 1–5 mSv when using specific iterative dose reduction techniques in CT scans) and the discomfort of ingesting a considerable amount of contrast liquid. Recently, dual-energy CT scan has been used in the evaluation of CD, with slightly better diagnostic accuracy than conventional CT [47]. Despite these technical improvements, recent studies have demonstrated [48].

Nevertheless, CT still provides higher sensitivity in detecting lymphadenopathies and in assessing the extent of abscesses and to plan their percutaneous drainages. Despite the overall accuracy of detecting active inflammation is comparable to MRIs, CT is no more considered as the reference imaging method in the initial diagnosis or to rule out CD complications. The rationale of CT is still to be found, however, in its favorable ratio between rapidity and diagnostic accuracy and in its wide availability, which makes it the best option in the emergency setting [49].

7.7 Nuclear Medicine

In severe CD cases, a 18FDG-PET/CT hybrid imaging may be useful for the evaluation of CD as it is highly sensitive in identifying acute inflammation, even more than MRI in some recent published studies [32, 50]. FDG-PET/CT combined with ultrasound resulted in a 100% detection rate of strictures in a recent work by Lenze et al. [32, 50]. Also, a hybrid approach has been found useful in discriminating between purely fibrotic, acute inflammatory, and mixed strictures. Imaging biomarkers extracted from PET/MRI images like SUVmax, signal intensity on T2-weighted images × SUVmax and ADC × SUVmax [51]. In particular, ADC × SUVmax > 3000 is the indicated threshold to differentiate purely fibrotic strictures from inflammatory or mixed ones.

7.8 Future Prospects

State-of-the-art CD imaging allows to noninvasively monitor disease activity and treatment response (Fig. 7.5).

Latest efforts aim to provide functional information about disease activity in order to achieve an earlier diagnosis. MRI-based investigations are focusing on

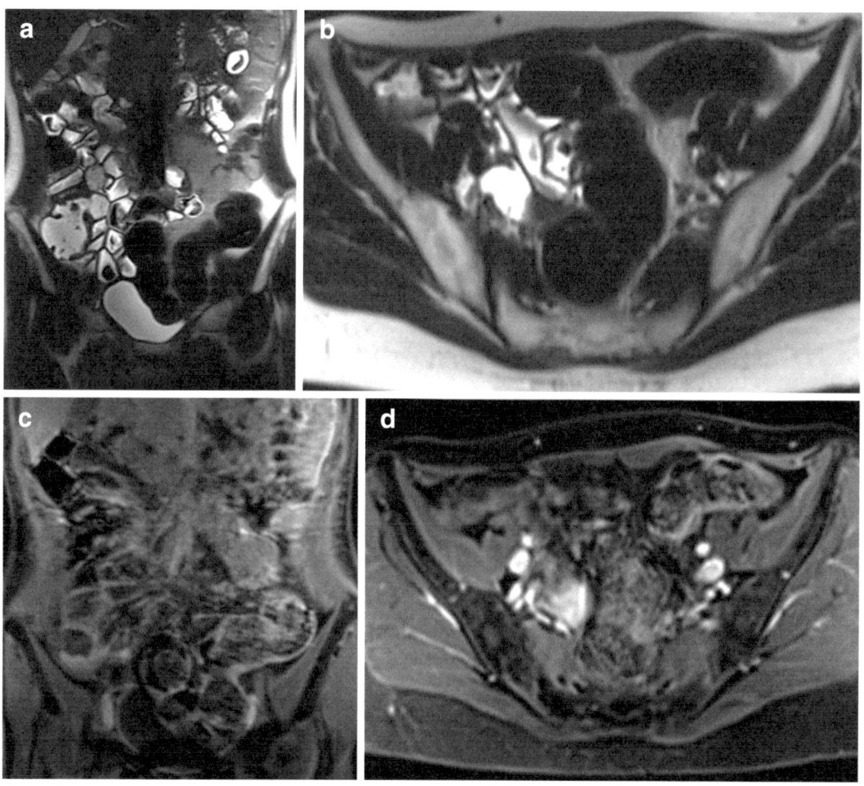

Fig. 7.5 Same patient of Fig. 7.1 (**a**) T2-W sequence in coronal and axial plane (**b**) shows resolution of the strictures and of the inflammatory parameters after therapy. T1-W FS sequence after Gd administration shows only mild wall enhancement

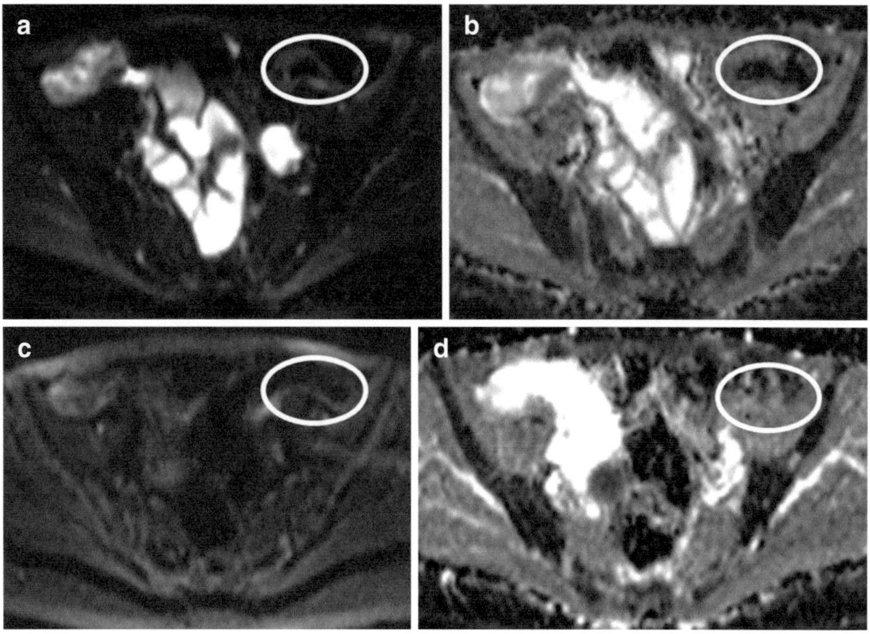

Fig. 7.6 (**a**) DWI ($b = 800$) shows high signal intensity in a proximal sigmoid tract with correspondent ADC restriction (**b**). (**c**) Axial DWI ($b = 800$) shows no areas of high signal intensity with no restriction in the ADC map (**d**) after therapy

interesting technologies like the MR diffusion-weighted imaging and MR magnetization transfer imaging. DW imaging promises to detect early inflammatory changes or early treatment response (Fig. 7.6).

DWI hyperintensity correlated well with endoscopic inflammation in CD and may play a critical role in the assessment of patients who cannot bear IV contrast administration. MR magnetization transfer imaging rose excitement about its potential ability to discriminate fibrotic scarring from acute inflammation by quantifying the mean magnetization transfer ratio, which is lower in tissues with active inflammation [38]. Fast cinematic balanced steady-state free precession sequences are another frontier that needs to be further investigated. In addition to this traditional protocol, newer MRI techniques have been introduced in the study of CD, like the automated motility mapping analysis and magnetization transfer MR. As peristalsis functionality is compromised in CD, its evaluation through particular MRI sequences is useful to quantify its involvement. Sequences like fast T2-W SSFP or echo planar with serial acquisition of images every 300–1000 ms during a normal breath-hold period can assess visually and quantitatively if the normal peristalsis is still preserved. One last point has to be dedicated to hybrid imaging. As a raising imaging modality, MRI can be coupled with a simultaneous positron-emission tomography acquisition. The PET/MRI scan combines an excellent morphologic portrait of the pathology with the pharmacokinetic functional information of PET. No strong evidence have been presented yet, but the growing interest in the hybrid approach will provide soon more insights [52]. Ultrasound elastography imaging (UEI) is an emerging imaging technique which has already showed promising results [53] in detecting bowel fibrosis in advanced CD. Further validation is needed to guide UEI into the daily clinical practice.

Endoscopy is not well accepted by most patients, and an alternative, noninvasive method to assess mucosal healing would be appreciated. MRI has shown promising results with the introduction of the magnetic resonance index of activity (MaRIA), which correlated well with endoscopic findings [54]. Novel MR biomarkers could represent the logical next step toward accurate assessment of bowel mucosa.

In conclusion, the efforts of modern imaging aim to provide a meticulous monitoring program of the disease progression and of the early treatment response, in order to improve the long-term outcome and to prevent irreversible structural damage.

References

1. Freeman HJ. Natural history and clinical behavior of Crohn's disease extending beyond two decades. J Clin Gastroenterol. 2003;37:216–9.
2. Sasaki T, Kunisaki R, Kinoshita H, et al. Doppler ultrasound findings correlate with tissue vascularity and inflammation in surgical pathology specimens from patients with small intestinal Crohn's disease. BMC Res Notes. 2014;7:363.
3. Dignass A, Van Assche G, Lindsay JO, et al. The second European evidence-based consensus on the diagnosis and management of Crohn's disease: current management. J Crohns Colitis. 2010;4:28–62.
4. Yamamoto T. Factors affecting recurrence after surgery for Crohn's disease. World J Gastroenterol. 2005;11:3971–9.
5. Peyrin-Biroulet L, Cieza A, Sandborn WJ, et al. Development of the first disability index for inflammatory bowel disease based on the international classification of functioning, disability and health. Gut. 2012;61:241–7.
6. Gasche C, Scholmerich J, Brynskov J, et al. A simple classification of Crohn's disease: report of the Working Party for the World Congresses of Gastroenterology, Vienna 1998. Inflamm Bowel Dis. 2000;6:8–15.
7. Louis E, Collard A, Oger AF, et al. Behaviour of Crohn's disease according to the Vienna classification: changing pattern over the course of the disease. Gut. 2001;49:777–82.
8. Cosnes J, Cattan S, Blain A, et al. Long-term evolution of disease behavior of Crohn's disease. Inflamm Bowel Dis. 2002;8:244–50.
9. Molenaar ETH, Voskuyl AE, Dinant HJ, et al. Progression of radiologic damage in patients with rheumatoid arthritis in clinical remission. Arthritis Rheum. 2004;50:36–42.
10. Danese S, Fiorino G, Peyrin-Biroulet L. Early intervention in Crohn's disease: towards disease modification trials. Gut. 2017;66:2179–87.
11. Ordás I, Rimola J, Rodríguez S, et al. Accuracy of magnetic resonance enterography in assessing response to therapy and mucosal healing in patients with Crohn's disease. Gastroenterology. 2014;146:374–82.e1.
12. Fiorino G, Bonifacio C, Allocca M, et al. Bowel damage as assessed by the Lémann index is reversible on anti-TNF therapy for Crohn's disease. J Crohns Colitis. 2015;9:633–9.
13. Bodini G, Giannini EG, De Maria C, et al. Anti-TNF therapy is able to stabilize bowel damage progression in patients with Crohn's disease. A study performed using the Lémann index. Dig Liver Dis. 2017;49:175–80.

14. Fiorino G, Morin M, Bonovas S, et al. Prevalence of bowel damage assessed by cross-sectional imaging in early Crohn's disease and its impact on disease outcome. J Crohns Colitis. 2017;11:274–80.
15. Peyrin-Biroulet L, Loftus EV, Colombel J-F, et al. Early Crohn disease: a proposed definition for use in disease-modification trials. Gut. 2010;59:141–7.
16. Fiorino G, Bonifacio C, Peyrin-Biroulet L, et al. Preventing collateral damage in Crohn's disease: the Lémann index. J Crohns Colitis. 2016;10:495–500.
17. Silverberg MS, Satsangi J, Ahmad T, et al. Toward an integrated clinical, molecular and serological classification of inflammatory bowel disease: report of a Working Party of the 2005 Montreal World Congress of Gastroenterology. Can J Gastroenterol. 2005;19(Suppl A):5A–36A.
18. Vester-Andersen MK, Prosberg MV, Jess T, et al. Disease course and surgery rates in inflammatory bowel disease: a population-based, 7-year follow-up study in the era of immunomodulating therapy. Am J Gastroenterol. 2014;109:705–14.
19. Panés J, Bouzas R, Chaparro M, et al. Systematic review: the use of ultrasonography, computed tomography and magnetic resonance imaging for the diagnosis, assessment of activity and abdominal complications of Crohn's disease. Aliment Pharmacol Ther. 2011;34:125–45.
20. Pariente B, Peyrin-Biroulet L, Cohen L, et al. Gastroenterology review and perspective: the role of cross-sectional imaging in evaluating bowel damage in Crohn disease. AJR Am J Roentgenol. 2011;197:42–9.
21. Fiorino G, Bonifacio C, Peyrin-Biroulet L, et al. Prospective comparison of computed tomography enterography and magnetic resonance enterography for assessment of disease activity and complications in ileocolonic Crohn's disease. Inflamm Bowel Dis. 2011;17:1073–80.
22. Daperno M, D'Haens G, Van Assche G, et al. Development and validation of a new, simplified endoscopic activity score for Crohn's disease: the SES-CD. Gastrointest Endosc. 2004;60:505–12.
23. Mary JY, Modigliani R. Development and validation of an endoscopic index of the severity for Crohn's disease: a prospective multicentre study. Groupe d'Etudes Thérapeutiques des Affections Inflammatoires du Tube Digestif (GETAID). Gut. 1989;30:983–9.
24. Pariente B, Mary J-Y, Danese S, et al. Development of the Lémann index to assess digestive tract damage in patients with Crohn's disease. Gastroenterology. 2015;148:52–63.e3.
25. Rimola J, Rodriguez S, García-Bosch O, et al. Magnetic resonance for assessment of disease activity and severity in ileocolonic Crohn's disease. Gut. 2009;58:1113–20.
26. Eder P, Michalak M, Katulska K, et al. Magnetic resonance enterographic predictors of one-year outcome in ileal and ileocolonic Crohn's disease treated with anti-tumor necrosis factor antibodies. Sci Rep. 2015;5:10223.
27. Tielbeek JAW, Ziech MLW, Li Z, et al. Evaluation of conventional, dynamic contrast enhanced and diffusion weighted MRI for quantitative Crohn's disease assessment with histopathology of surgical specimens. Eur Radiol. 2014;24:619–29.
28. Punwani S, Rodriguez-Justo M, Bainbridge A, et al. Mural inflammation in Crohn disease: location-matched histologic validation of MR imaging features. Radiology. 2009;252:712–20.
29. Zappa M, Stefanescu C, Cazals-Hatem D, et al. Which magnetic resonance imaging findings accurately evaluate inflammation in small bowel Crohn's disease? A retrospective comparison with surgical pathologic analysis. Inflamm Bowel Dis. 2011;17:984–93.
30. Adler J, Punglia DR, Dillman JR, et al. Computed tomography enterography findings correlate with tissue inflammation, not fibrosis in resected small bowel Crohn's disease. Inflamm Bowel Dis. 2012;18:849–56.
31. Rieder F, Fiocchi C. Intestinal fibrosis in IBD—a dynamic, multifactorial process. Nat Rev Gastroenterol Hepatol. 2009;6:228–35.
32. Lenze F, Wessling J, Bremer J, et al. Detection and differentiation of inflammatory versus fibromatous Crohn's disease strictures: prospective comparison of 18F-FDG-PET/CT, MR-enteroclysis, and transabdominal ultrasound versus endoscopic/histologic evaluation. Inflamm Bowel Dis. 2012;18:2252–60.

33. Latella G, Sferra R, Speca S, et al. Can we prevent, reduce or reverse intestinal fibrosis in IBD? Eur Rev Med Pharmacol Sci. 2013;17:1283–304.
34. Lahat A, Chowers Y. The patient with recurrent (sub) obstruction due to Crohn's disease. Best Pract Res Clin Gastroenterol. 2007;21:427–44.
35. Van Assche G, Geboes K, Rutgeerts P. Medical therapy for Crohn's disease strictures. Inflamm Bowel Dis. 2004;10:55–60.
36. Ram R, Sarver D, Pandey T, et al. Magnetic resonance enterography: a stepwise interpretation approach and role of imaging in management of adult Crohn's disease. Indian J Radiol Imaging. 2016;26:173–84.
37. Satsangi J, Silverberg MS, Vermeire S, et al. The Montreal classification of inflammatory bowel disease: controversies, consensus, and implications. Gut. 2006;55:749–53.
38. Fiorino G, Bonifacio C, Malesci A, et al. MRI in Crohn's disease—current and future clinical applications. Nat Rev Gastroenterol Hepatol. 2011;9:23–31.
39. Rimola J, Planell N, Rodríguez S, et al. Characterization of inflammation and fibrosis in Crohn's disease lesions by magnetic resonance imaging. Am J Gastroenterol. 2015;110:432–40.
40. Ripollés T, Rausell N, Paredes JM, et al. Effectiveness of contrast-enhanced ultrasound for characterisation of intestinal inflammation in Crohn's disease: a comparison with surgical histopathology analysis. J Crohns Colitis. 2013;7:120–8.
41. Wilkens R, Peters DA, Nielsen AH, et al. Dynamic contrast-enhanced magnetic resonance enterography and dynamic contrast-enhanced ultrasonography in Crohn's disease: an observational comparison study. Ultrasound Int Open. 2017;3:E13–24.
42. Morimoto K, Watanabe K, Noguchi A, et al. Clinical impact of ultrathin colonoscopy for Crohn's disease patients with strictures. J Gastroenterol Hepatol. 2015;30(Suppl 1):66–70.
43. Fraquelli M, Branchi F, Cribiù FM, et al. The role of ultrasound elasticity imaging in predicting ileal fibrosis in Crohn's disease patients. Inflamm Bowel Dis. 2015;21:2605–12.
44. Dillman JR, Stidham RW, Higgins PDR, et al. Ultrasound shear wave elastography helps discriminate low-grade from high-grade bowel wall fibrosis in ex vivo human intestinal specimens. J Ultrasound Med. 2014;33:2115–23.
45. Calabrese E, Zorzi F, Zuzzi S, et al. Development of a numerical index quantitating small bowel damage as detected by ultrasonography in Crohn's disease. J Crohns Colitis. 2012;6:852–60.
46. Calabrese E, Zorzi F, Pallone F. Ultrasound of the small bowel in Crohn's disease. Int J Inflam. 2012;2012:964720.
47. Peng JC, Feng Q, Zhu J, et al. Usefulness of spectral computed tomography for evaluation of intestinal activity and severity in ileocolonic Crohn's disease. Therap Adv Gastroenterol. 2016;9:795–805.
48. Panes J, Bouhnik Y, Reinisch W, et al. Imaging techniques for assessment of inflammatory bowel disease: joint ECCO and ESGAR evidence-based consensus guidelines. J Crohns Colitis. 2013;7:556–85.
49. Haas K, Rubesova E, Bass D. Role of imaging in the evaluation of inflammatory bowel disease: how much is too much? World J Radiol. 2016;8:124–31.
50. Holtmann MH, Uenzen M, Helisch A, et al. 18F-Fluorodeoxyglucose positron-emission tomography (PET) can be used to assess inflammation non-invasively in Crohn's disease. Dig Dis Sci. 2012;57:2658–68.
51. Catalano OA, et al. Evaluation of quantitative PET/MR enterography biomarkers for discrimination of inflammatory strictures from fibrotic strictures in crohn disease. Radiology. 2016;278:792–800. https://doi.org/10.1148/radiol.2015150566.
52. Stanley E, Moriarty HK, Cronin CG. Advanced multimodality imaging of inflammatory bowel disease in 2015: an update. World J Radiol. 2016;8:571–80.
53. Giannetti A, Matergi M, Biscontri M, et al. Real-time elastography in Crohn's disease: feasibility in daily clinical practice. J Ultrasound. 2017;20:147–55.
54. Buisson A, Pereira B, Goutte M, et al. Magnetic resonance index of activity (MaRIA) and Clermont score are highly and equally effective MRI indices in detecting mucosal healing in Crohn's disease. Dig Liver Dis. 2017;49:1211–7.

MRI of Perianal Crohn's Disease

8

Kyra L. van Rijn and Jaap Stoker

Abstract

Perianal disease is a common complication in Crohn's disease and imaging helps the clinician in the diagnosis and decisions regarding therapeutic strategy. Pelvic MRI is the recommended imaging modality because of its accuracy and advantages compared to other imaging techniques. Specific sequences and planes are mandatory for adequate assessment of perianal Crohn's disease. It is important to understand the perianal anatomy to adequately describe the anatomical location and extension of fistula. Other aspects in the assessment of perianal disease on MRI include the assessment of fistula activity, presence of abscesses and proctitis, and assessment of response to therapy. This chapter provides an overview of technical MRI features, pelvic anatomy, and different aspects of perianal Crohn's disease on MRI for an adequate diagnostic workup.

8.1 Introduction Perianal Crohn's Disease

Perianal fistulas are a common complication in Crohn's disease; about 13–27% of patients develop perianal fistulas during the course of their disease with an estimated cumulative risk of 26–28% after 20 years and a recurrence in 34% of patients. In around 17% of patients with perianal Crohn's disease, perianal fistula is the initial presentation [1, 2].

K. L. van Rijn (✉) · J. Stoker
Department of Radiology and Nuclear Medicine, Amsterdam UMC, University of Amsterdam, Amsterdam, The Netherlands
e-mail: k.l.vanrijn@amc.uva.nl; j.stoker@amc.uva.nl

J. Rimola (ed.), *Cross-Sectional Imaging in Crohn's Disease*,
https://doi.org/10.1007/978-3-319-96586-4_8

The diagnosis of perianal fistula is based on clinical findings and imaging. Important aspects in the evaluation of perianal fistula are the anatomic classification, assessment of activity, and description of response to therapy [3–5].

Several guidelines, among which global and European guidelines, state that MRI is the first choice in diagnostic modalities for the assessment of perianal Crohn's disease because it is highly accurate and noninvasive [3–6].

MRI has impact on the course of treatment, regarding choices for surgical interventions and/or drug therapy. Drug therapy consists of biologicals, sometimes combined with other immunosuppressants and/or antibiotics. Surgical interventions are initially focused on drainage of abscesses and placement of setons to keep tracts open for drainage, controlling the inflammation while the patient is under biological treatment and, in selected cases, in later stadia on more definitive surgical procedures, for example, closing the internal opening with a mucosal advancement flap (MAF procedure) or ligation and transection of a fistula tract via an intersphincteric approach (LIFT procedure).

8.2 MRI Versus Other Diagnostic Modalities

Other imaging modalities in the evaluation of perianal Crohn's disease are endoanal ultrasound (EUS), perineal ultrasound, and an examination under anesthesia (EUA).

Endoanal ultrasound uses an internal transducer and is accurate for the visualization of internal openings and tracks close to the anal canal; however, disadvantages are a limited field of view for more extended fistula tracts and invasiveness restricting its use to patients without anal strictures. Perineal ultrasound is a less-invasive alternative but also has a limited depth penetration resulting in inadequate visualization of more extended tracts and abscesses. It could have a benefit in the detection of anovaginal tracts.

A prospective study comparing endoanal ultrasound, MRI, and exam under anesthesia reported accuracies of 91%, 87%, and 91%, respectively, and when any two techniques were combined, a 100% accuracy was reached [7]. Another large prospective study showed that the accuracy of MRI exceeded that of endoanal ultrasound and digital examination in the classification of fistulas (90%, 81%, 61%, respectively) [8]. Comparable sensitivities for MRI and endoanal ultrasound (both 87%) were shown in a meta-analysis but with a higher specificity for MRI (69% vs. 43%) [9]. Perineal ultrasound has not been studied extensively; one study showed correct detection and anatomical classification of fistulas with a sensitivity of 89%, but abscesses with a sensitivity of only 50%, resulting in a combined correct detection and classification in 67% of patients [10].

Advantages of MRI compared to other imaging techniques are the noninvasive character, overview, and intrinsic contrast resolution. MRI is able to assess the entire perianal region and pelvic floor (and beyond) including extensive tracts as well as abscesses and proctitis. Alternatively, endoanal ultrasound can be used for assessment of perianal disease.

8.3 Anatomy

It is important to understand the anal and perianal anatomy for the assessment of perianal disease on MRI.

The anal anatomy is—in its basic form—straightforward, namely, a few cylindrical structures, from inside out: epithelium and subepithelium (mucosa/submucosa with muscularis mucosae), internal sphincter, intersphincteric space, and outermost striated muscle (lower-half external sphincter and upper-half puborectal muscle (Fig. 8.1)).

The anorectal canal is covered by epithelium, the most distal two centimeters by squamous epithelium that turns into columnar epithelium at a transition zone, the dentate line (not visible at imaging). At this transition zone lie the crypts of Morgagni with the anal glands. There are two hypotheses regarding the etiology of perianal fistulas, one is the infection of these anal glands which is the cryptoglandular hypothesis and applies to patients without Crohn's disease and may play a role in Crohn's disease as well [11]. The second hypothesis is that in Crohn's disease, fistula tracts originate from penetrating ulcerations within the anorectal canal [12].

The internal sphincter consists of smooth muscle and is an extension of the inner circular muscle layer of the rectum. The intersphincteric space contains fat, connective tissue, and the longitudinal layer (continuation of the longitudinal muscle of the rectal wall). The width of the intersphincteric space varies between individuals (can be slit like and hard to discern on imaging in some) and is also called intersphincteric plane.

The external sphincter consists of striated muscle and can be subdivided in a deep part, a superficial part and a subcutaneous part; these subdivisions are to a variable extent recognizable at imaging. Cranial to the external sphincter is the puborectal muscle (i.e., is the upper half of the outer anal sphincter), which is a sling that is anteriorly open with attachment to the pubic bone at each side.

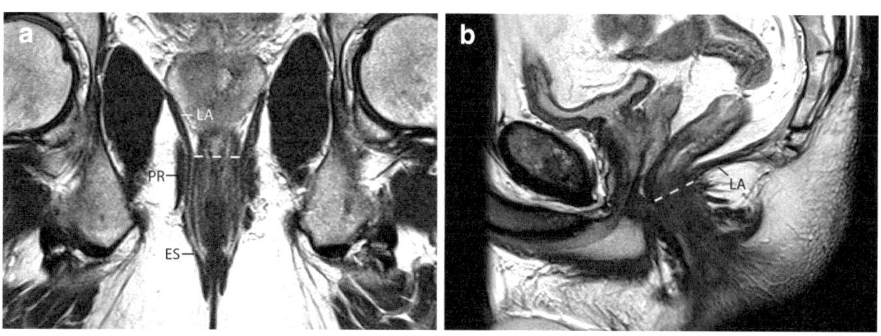

Fig. 8.1 Normal anatomy on oblique coronal (**a**) and sagittal (**b**) T2-weighted sequences, pointed out are the external sphincter (ES), puborectal muscle (PR), and levator ani muscle (LA). The white dashed line represents the anorectal junction, at the transition of the superior border of the puborectal muscle to the levator ani muscle

Muscles closely aligned to the anal sphincter include the bulbospongiosus muscle and transverse perineal muscle anteriorly and the pelvic diaphragm superiorly including the levator plate with pubococcygeus muscle and iliococcygeus muscle (both part of the levator ani muscle).

The anus is continuous with the rectum, and the anorectal junction lies at the transition of the superior border of the puborectal muscle to the levator ani muscle bordering the hiatus. On pelvic MRI, the anorectal junction is most easily recognized on sagittal and coronal sequences, as the levator ani (iliococcygeus part) on a coronal sequence extends laterally and cranial towards the pelvic wall on both sides and on a sagittal sequence the levator ani (pubococcygeus part) posteriorly extends to the coccyx (Fig. 8.1). On axial sequences, visualization of the anorectal junction is not reached in one plane; it is at the level where there is the change from the cylindrical structures of the anal sphincter to lateral fanning out of the pelvic floor muscles when scrolling upward through the images (or vice versa when scrolling downward).

The anal sphincter is surrounded by the ischioanal space (also named ischiorectal space) and perineum (antero) inferiorly and contains mostly fat.

8.4 MRI Technique for Perianal Crohn's Disease

MRI of perianal fistulas is performed with phased-array surface coils at either 1.5 or 3.0 T (see Table 8.1, examples of MRI protocols). Although endoluminal coils can be used, the field of view is limited by signal drop-off caused by the small effective volume of the endoanal coil (Fig. 8.2.). Especially in Crohn's patients, where tracks can extend substantially outside the anal sphincter, this can be a limitation. Together with their limited availability, this narrows their use in clinical practice [13]. Endoanal coils could have a benefit in visualization of the more difficult ano- or rectovaginal fistulas and for visualizing subtle internal openings because of the local higher spatial resolution [14, 15] (Fig. 8.2).

8.4.1 Sequences

A T2-weighted sequence is most adequate in visualizing the pelvic anatomy, showing sufficient contrast between the different sphincter components and fistula. The sequence should be more toward proton-density weighting than strong T2 weighting for better visualization and discrimination of the different anatomical structures, which help for fistula classification (identification of fluid or granulation tissue is better with stronger T2 weighting, but the use of a fat-sat sequence precludes the need for stronger T2 weighting). The external sphincter and puborectal muscle (and other striated muscles) are relatively hypointense. The internal sphincter is hyperintense compared to the external sphincter on T2-weighted sequences and has a homogeneous structure.

For the assessment of fistulas, an additional T2-weighted sequence with fat suppression is mandatory as it helps in identifying and assessing the fistula tract and

Table 8.1 Example of scan protocols at different field strengths with external phased-array coils

	Sagittal T2-weighted turbo spin-echo	Coronal T2-weighted turbo spin-echo	Axial T2-weighted turbo spin-echo	Axial T2-weighted turbo spin-echo with fat suppression	Axial T1-weighted turbo spin-echo with fat saturation after IV contrast administration
(a) 1.5 T MRI scanner					
TE (ms)	70	70	70	70	9.4
TR (ms)	2500	2500	2500	2500	600
Turbo factor	11	11	11	3	3
Averages	2	2	2	2	3
Field of view (mm)	300	300	300	300	300
Slice thickness (mm)	4	4	4	4	4
Pixel size (mm)	0.8 × 0.6	0.8 × 0.6	0.8 × 0.6	0.8 × 0.6	1.3 × 0.9
(b) 3.0 T MRI scanner					
TE (ms)	60	60	60	60	8
TR (ms)	2500–3000	2500–3000	2500–3000	2500–3000	650
Turbo factor	20	20	20	20	8
Averages	1	1	1	1	1
Field of view (mm)	240	240	240	240	240
Slice thickness (mm)	3	3	3	3	3
Pixel size (mm)	0.6 × 0.7	0.6 × 0.7	0.6 × 0.7	0.6 × 0.7	0.6 × 0.7

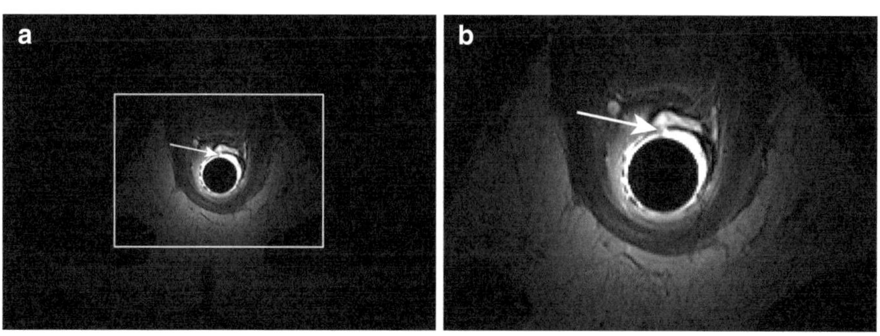

Fig. 8.2 MRI with endoluminal coil showing the small field of view with signal drop-off (**a**) but also the advantage in visualizing the internal opening of a fistula tract (*arrow*) (**b**)

distinguishing fluid and fat. A STIR sequence might be an alternative to a T2-weighted fat-suppressed sequence, although the detail might be somewhat less than for a fat-saturated T2-weighted sequence [16].

A T1-weighted axial sequence after intravenous administration of a gadolinium-based contrast agent is recommended for the assessment of fistula activity and is important for distinguishing fluid from granulation tissue (Figs. 8.3 and 8.4).

A spasmolytic agent is not routinely used. When endoluminal MRI is used, a spasmolytic agent is strongly recommended to reduce artifacts by bowel peristalsis.

8.4.2 MRI Planes

1. Sagittal T2-weighted sequence. This sequence is performed first as it is also used to set the following sequences referenced to the anal canal.
2. Oblique coronal T2-weighted sequence parallel to anal canal.

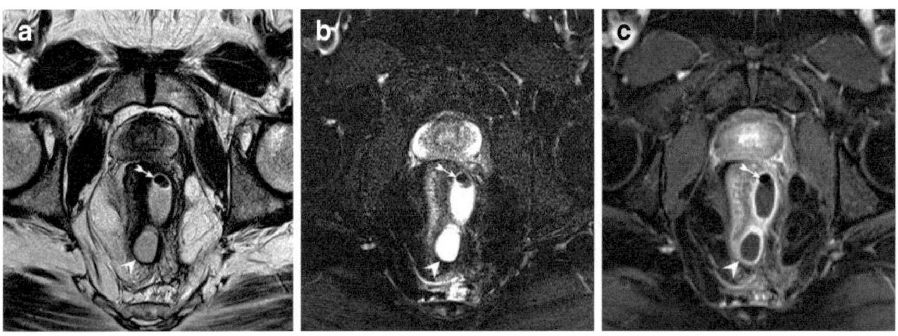

Fig. 8.3 An abscess (arrowhead) on axial oblique sequences: relatively hyperintense on a T2-weighted sequence (**a**), hyperintense on a T2-weighted sequence with fat suppression (**b**), and rim enhancement (i.e., granulation tissue) with a hypointense content (i.e., fluid) on a T1-weighted post-contrast sequence (**c**). On every sequence gas is visible anteriorly as a hypointense area in the abscess (tailed arrow)

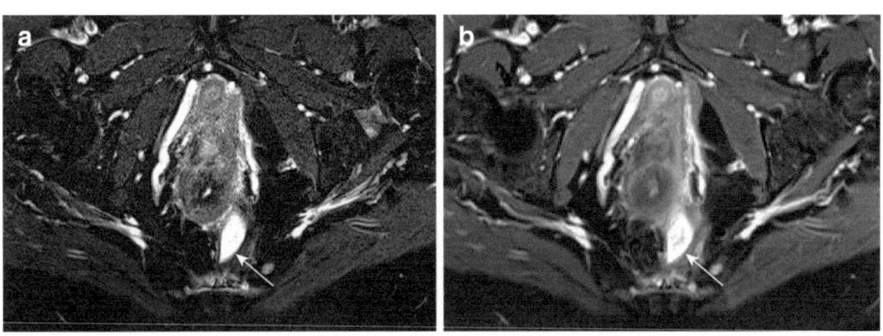

Fig. 8.4 Hyperintense collection (arrow) which can be interpreted as fluid or granulation tissue on a T2-weighted fat-suppressed sequence (**a**). The contrast-enhanced T1-weighted sequence (**b**) shows almost full enhancement indicating a circumscribed area with granulation tissue and very little fluid (compare to Fig. 8.3)

3. Oblique axial T2-weighted sequence without and with fat suppression and fat-saturated T1-weighted sequence after intravenous contrast administration perpendicular to the anal canal. It is important to have at least one slice inferior to the lower border of the anal sphincter and several slices above the anorectal junction (otherwise for proctitis evaluation, only sagittal and coronal T2-weighted sequences are available).

8.4.3 Novel Sequences

Over the last years, novel sequences have been tested in patients with perianal Crohn's disease which could play an additional role in evaluation, but their use in clinical practice has not been firmly established.

8.4.3.1 Diffusion-Weighted Imaging (DWI)

DWI is a MRI technique using differences in the diffusion of water molecules and is hereby able to reflect information on (among others) inflammatory activity. A study by Dohan et al. showed that DWI (b-values 0, 600 and 1000 s/mm^2) is accurate in the detection of abscesses and can differentiate between an abscess with pus and collection with granulation tissue [17]. A retrospective study of Hori et al. showed an additional value of DWI (b-values 0 and 800 s/mm^2) compared to T2-weighted sequences alone and in a small sample ($n = 13$) with a similar accuracy to (fat-suppressed) T1-weighted imaging with contrast enhancement [18]. There is until now too limited data to support DWI replacing (fat-suppressed) T1-weighted imaging after contrast medium, but in clinical practice DWI can be considered in patients unable to receive intravenous contrast agents.

8.4.3.2 Dynamic Contrast-Enhanced Imaging (DCE)

DCE has the ability to quantitatively reflect tissue characteristics due to its dynamic evaluation of contrast agent inflow. DCE has been shown to have potential in the assessment of activity in perianal Crohn's disease [19]. Preliminary data also showed that it could be an indicator of early response to therapy [20]. The technique could be promising, but more research is needed to evaluate its clinical value.

8.4.3.3 Magnetization Transfer (MT)

A very recent topic is magnetization-transfer MRI for perianal fistulas, which showed to be feasible to distinguish active from inactive fistulas. The technique should be studied further before conclusions on its clinical applicability can be drawn [21].

8.5 Assessment of Perianal Crohn's Disease on MRI

8.5.1 Perianal Fistula

A fistula is an abnormal tract that connects two epithelial surfaces. Perianal fistula in Crohn's disease mostly begin in the anal canal and extend to the perineal skin, but also other types of tracts, like anovaginal tracts, can occur (Fig. 8.5). In Crohn's

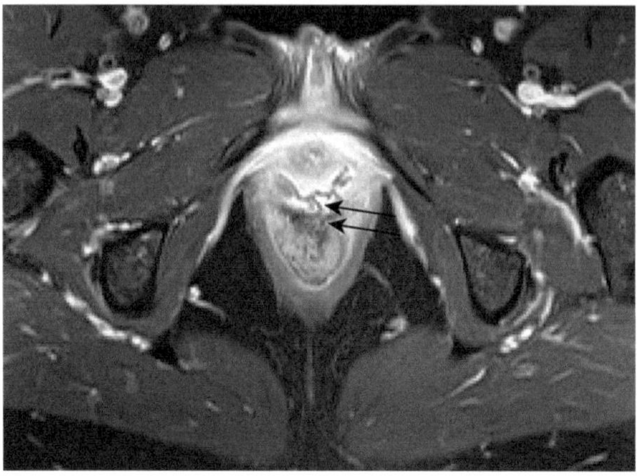

Fig. 8.5 Anovaginal fistula (arrows) at an oblique axial T1-weighted post-contrast sequence with fat saturation

disease extensive perianal disease is not uncommon, which is very uncommon in perianal fistula related to cryptoglandular disease. In a patient with extensive perianal fistula disease and no previous history of Crohn's disease, the diagnosis of perianal Crohn's disease should be considered.

Description of the anatomic location, extension, and disease activity are important in the assessment of perianal fistula and have implications for treatment and prognosis.

8.5.1.1 Anatomic Location and Extension

The location of perianal fistula is basically described in relation to the internal sphincter and external sphincter/puborectal muscle. Mostly the modified Park's classification is used [22] in which fistulae can be classified as submucosal or inter-, trans-, extra-, or suprasphincteric. A submucosal fistula tract is superficial to the internal sphincter and does not involve any part of the sphincter muscles (this track was not defined in the original publication by Parks). An intersphincteric fistula tract runs from the anal canal through the internal sphincter into the intersphincteric space and then downward, ending at the perineal skin (it does not transverse the outer striated muscle layer of external sphincter and puborectal muscle) (Fig. 8.6). A transsphincteric fistula develops from the anal canal into the intersphincteric space and then crosses the outer striated muscle layer which can occur at any level so either through the external sphincter or the puborectal muscle (Figs. 8.7 and 8.8). A suprasphincteric tract transverses the internal sphincter into the intersphincteric plane and then goes up above the level of the anorectal junction (i.e., above the superior border of the puborectal muscle) and down through the levator plate into the ischioanal fossa and perineal skin. An extrasphincteric tract runs from the rectal epithelium to the levator plate, ischioanal fossa, and then to the perineal skin; this track has no involvement of the anal sphincter.

The most common tracts in patients referred for MRI are intersphincteric and transsphincteric; other tracts are relatively rare findings. An extrasphincteric tract exclusively develops after prior perianal disease, mostly after surgery.

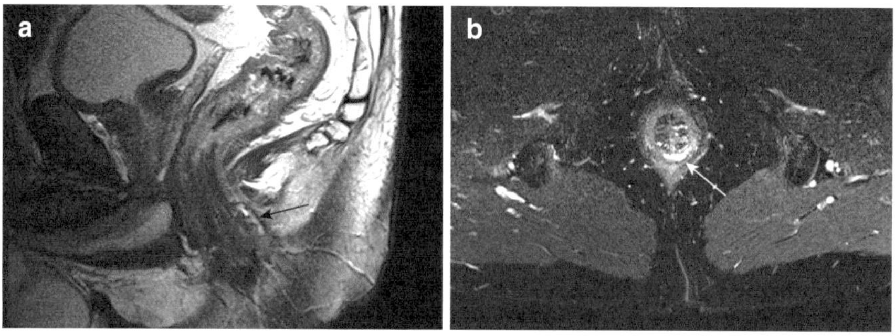

Fig. 8.6 An intersphincteric tract (arrow) on a sagittal T2-weighted sequence (**a**) and oblique axial T2-weighted fat-suppressed sequence (**b**)

Fig. 8.7 T2-weighted sagittal sequence showing a low transsphincteric fistula coursing through the lower edge of the external sphincter (arrows)

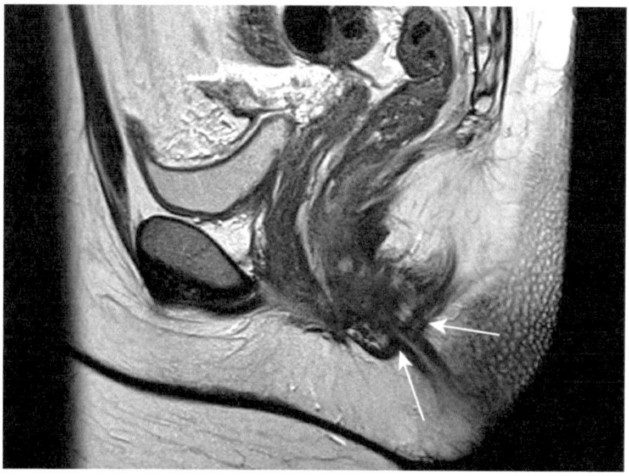

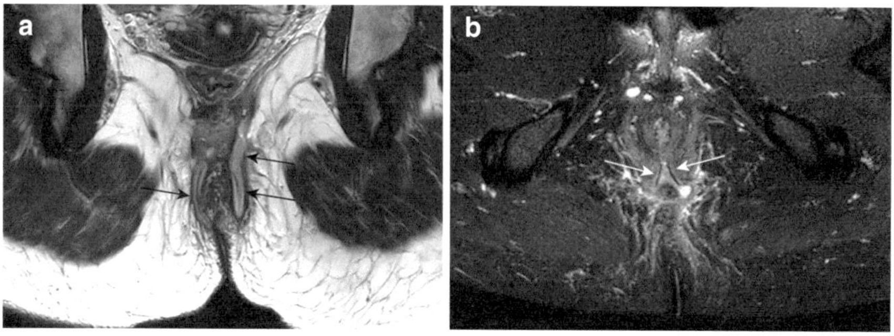

Fig. 8.8 Transsphincteric fistula tracts (arrows) with setons (hypointense lines in the tracts on a coronal T2-weighted sequence (**a**) and fat-suppressed axial oblique T2-weighted sequence (**b**)

The extension of the fistula tracts can be described in different ways. Samaan et al. divided fistulas in single and unbranched, single and branched, and complex and the extension as infralevatoric, supralevatoric, or horseshoe configuration, which is an intersphincteric extension around the internal sphincter filled with fluid and/or granulation tissue [23].

Another used distinction is in simple (e.g., single-branched submucosal, intersphincteric, or low transsphincteric fistula) and complex fistulas (e.g., fistulas that are not single-branched or located extrasphincteric, suprasphincteric, or anovaginal) [24].

Other anatomical classification systems exist, like the St. James University Hospital classification [25] that describes anatomical location, extension, and presence of abscesses in five grades. To our knowledge this system has not been widely adopted.

Which classification system to use will largely depend on the local situation; gastroenterologist, surgeon, and radiologist should use the same terminology and classification system. Often the modified Park's classification will be used, and certain additional features (e.g., abscesses) will be described. Advantages are that it is used for years and relatively simple. Although good for determining the extent of disease, this system does not systematically assess the full extent of disease and does not quantify disease activity (see Sect. 8.4.4 on fistula activity). Therefore it cannot be used for treatment monitoring such as the system proposed by Van Assche [26] or Samaan et al.; that system awaits further validation [23].

8.5.1.2 Location Internal Opening

Apart from the fistula classification, the location of the internal opening is important for a potential surgical intervention. The location of the internal opening in the axial plane can be described clockwise or be described based on the anatomical location in quadrants (e.g., anterior, right anterolateral, left posterolateral). When clockwise description is used, it should be clearly stated that anterior is 12 o'clock to prevent confusion depending whether surgical treatment is in supine or prone position.

The location of the internal opening in the longitudinal plane is described per half cm (or in mm) superior to the lowest border of the sphincter complex (i.e., external sphincter inferior border). Apart from the description in height as related to the lower sphincter border, it should be clear from the report where the track transverses the different sphincter structures, especially the outer striated muscles (external sphincter, puborectal muscle) in transsphincteric tracks. Additionally, it is an option to (also) report the distance of the internal opening to the anorectal junction; this is more important in high internal openings and depending on the preference of the clinician. As the length of the sphincter complex varies (mean women 56.6 ± 8.7 mm, men 55.5 ± 8.6 mm measured at endoanal MRI), only height measurements are insufficient to estimate the distance to the anorectal junction [27].

8.5.1.3 Fistula Activity

On a T2-weighted sequence (without and with fat suppression), an active fistula tract appears as hyperintense, while an inactive fibrous tract appears as

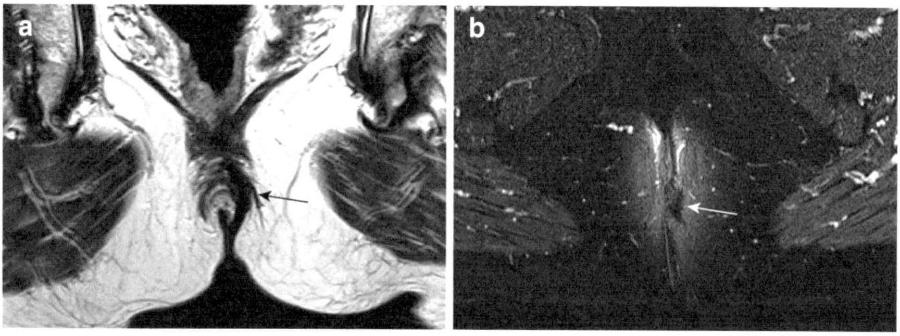

Fig. 8.9 A fistula (*arrow*) with hypointense signal intensity on an oblique coronal T2-weighted sequence (**a**) and oblique axial T2-weighted fat-suppressed sequence (**b**) indicates a fibrotic tract (the tract is also hypointense on a T1-weighted contrast-enhanced sequence but this is not shown here)

Fig. 8.10 A hypointense fibrous tract (*arrow*) on an oblique axial T2-weighted sequence (the tract is also hypointense on a T2-weighted sequence with fat suppression and T1-weighted contrast-enhanced sequence which are not shown here)

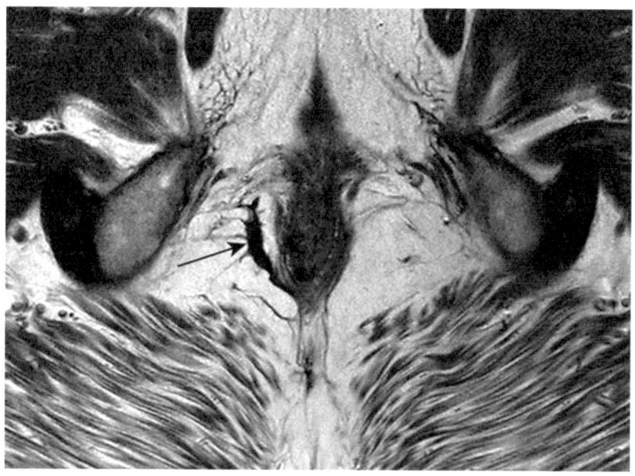

hypointense (Figs. 8.9 and 8.10). Some tracts are hypointense at the T2-weighted sequence but show some subtle hyperintensity at the fat-saturated T2-weighted sequence and fat-saturated T1-weighted contrast-enhanced sequence. These tracts have some remaining activity or reflect the gradual process to complete quiescent fibrous tissue. This can be discriminated by comparing sequential examinations and the intensity of the signal.

An active tract contains granulation tissue, fluid, or a combination. A track with only fluid and no granulation tissue will be rarely if ever encountered; a track is either completely obliterated by granulation tissue or has a central core of fluid (pus). The distinction between the predominant components can have implications for the course of treatment. Substantial fluid indicates inadequate drainage for which surgery is the best choice, while a mostly granulated tract may respond to drug therapy. A fat-saturated T1-weighted contrast-enhanced sequence will distinguish between the two; complete enhancement indicates granulation tissue, while a center of non-enhancement indicates fluid (pus).

8.5.2 Abscess

An abscess is a fluid collection that appears hyperintense on fat-saturated T2-weighted sequences, and on fat-saturated T1-weighted contrast-enhanced sequences, there is a typical pattern of rim enhancement (granulation tissue) with a hypointense center (fluid, i.e., pus) (Figs. 8.3 and 8.11). In some cases, there is no central fluid, and here it represents granulation tissue only (Fig. 8.4), which is an important difference for patient management. The definition of an abscess is not clearly established; a (locally) wider fistula tract with fluid can be interpreted as an abscess. In a classification by Van Assche (see Sect. 8.4.4 Treatment Response Monitoring), collections were described as cavities >3 mm [26]. Samaan et al. recently classified abscesses under the term inflammatory mass which includes diffuse inflammation (i.e., infiltrate), a focal lesion >3 mm with granulation tissue, and collections with rim enhancement divided in small (3–10 mm), medium (11–20 mm), and large (>20 mm) [23].

8.5.3 Proctitis

The inflammation of the rectum, proctitis, is another common finding in perianal Crohn's disease (Fig. 8.12). Its recognition is important because it has serious implications for the management and prognosis of fistulae [3]. The evaluation of proctitis on pelvic MRI is not completely similar to the evaluation of luminal disease on abdominal MRI because in pelvic MRI luminal contrast is not routinely performed and a smaller field of view is used. Tutein Nolthenius et al.

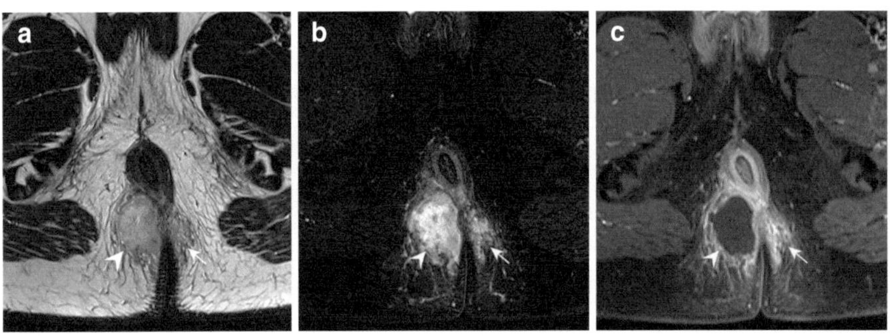

Fig. 8.11 Perianal abscess (arrowhead), heterogeneous relatively hyperintense on a T2-weighted oblique axial sequence (**a**), heterogeneous hyperintense on an oblique axial T2-weighted fat-suppressed sequence (**b**), and a typical hyperintense rim enhancement with hypointense content (fluid/pus) on an oblique axial T1-weighted contrast-enhanced sequence (**c**). The short arrow indicates inflammation in the surrounding fat tissue. MRI is often not indicated for superficial perianal abscesses; clinical examination is mostly sufficient to establish the need for drainage or if needed ultrasound or computed tomography can be performed in the acute setting. However, MRI can help in assessment of extension and course of additional fistula tracts and in some cases to establish the presence of an abscess

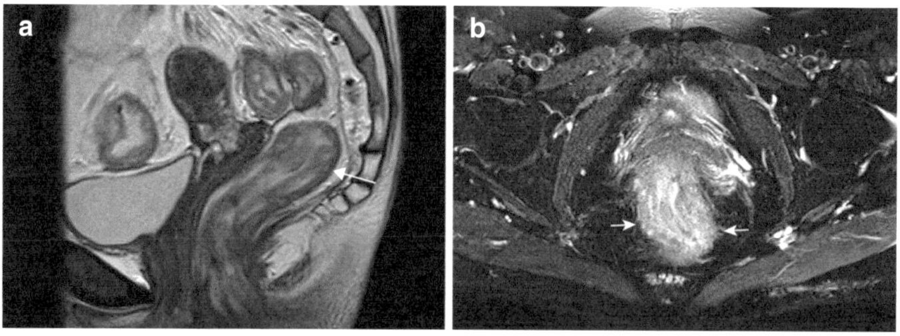

Fig. 8.12 Proctitis with wall thickening including abnormal stratification on a sagittal T2-weighted sequence (**a**) and perimural infiltration (short arrows) on an oblique axial fat-suppressed T2-weighted sequence (**b**). The T1 fat-suppressed contrast-enhanced sequence showed perimural enhancement (not shown here)

showed that MRI parameters that correlate to rectal inflammation on endoscopy are wall thickening, mural fat, and mesorectal features. The mesorectal features include perimural T2 sign, perimural enhancement, creeping fat, and size of mesorectal lymph nodes [28].

8.5.4 Treatment Response Monitoring

Therapy response assessment is based on clinical evaluation (mainly improvement of symptoms and closing of external openings) combined with imaging, but a validated index to measure response has not yet been established. MRI might be more feasible in the assessment of remission than clinical response; studies have shown that at clinical remission, tracts are often still active on MRI [26, 29]. This indicates that therapy should be continued after clinical remission has been reached, stopping drug therapy, while fistulas that remain active might have an impact on the recurrence of perianal fistula.

In the assessment of MRI for treatment response, several activity parameters should be evaluated. A decrease in signal intensity at a T2-weighted sequence, decreased enhancement, smaller volume, and limited extension are signs of response to therapy (Fig. 8.13). No change may indicate the need for a change of medical therapy.

In the need for a tool for the assessment of response to therapy, Van Assche et al. developed a score that includes anatomical features as described by Parks [22] as well as activity features consisting of the presence of T2 hyperintensity, extensions, abscesses, and proctitis. There was a certain weight given to the selected features based on expert opinion of these authors [26]. In their initial study, no significant difference was shown in baseline activity of responders versus nonresponders, but after 6 or 10 weeks of treatment, a greater decrease in activity was seen in the responding group [26]. One study showed that short-term response was related to a decrease in the Van Assche activity score but not a long-term response [30].

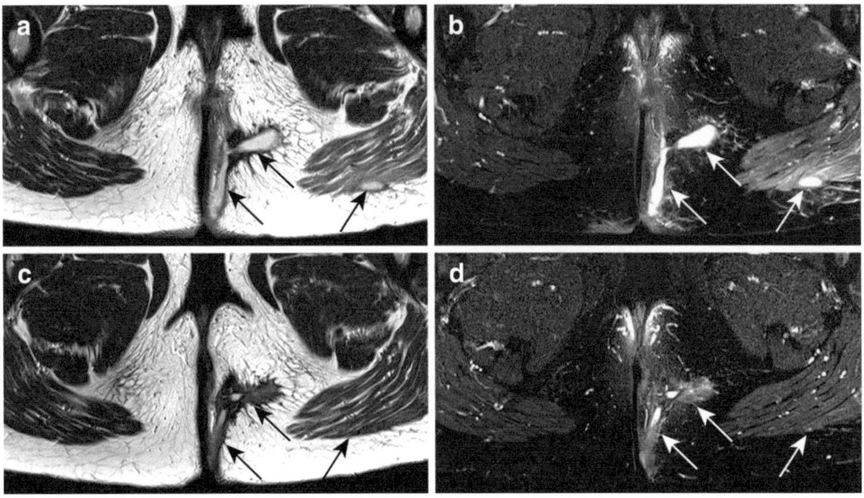

Fig. 8.13 Oblique axial T2-weighted sequences without (**a** and **c**) and with fat suppression (**b** and **d**) of a patient at baseline (**a** and **b**) and at follow-up (**c** and **d**), 21 months after initiation of drug therapy, illustrating a decrease in inflammatory activity of the fistula (*arrows*)

However, another study did not find a significant decrease in the Van Assche score in a group of clinically responders at 6, 12, and 18 months [29]. Horsthuis et al. added a T1-weighted contrast-enhanced sequence and presence of an infiltrate to the original Van Assche score, but no additional value was measured with regard to therapy response monitoring [31].

Recently, the Van Assche score was modified by an expert panel to improve the assessment of responsiveness to therapy and the inter- and intrarater reliability [23]. The scoring of certain items was adjusted, and several items were added to the original Van Assche score that were considered as features representing disease activity. Original items that were modified included the anatomical location where in the original score there was no submucosal tract included and extra- and intersphincteric were combined; in the new score, the locations as described by Parks with addition of the mucosal tract were all separate items. Also, in the original score, collections were described as absent or present, and in the modified score, this was adjusted to aspect of inflammatory mass including diffuse inflammation and different types and sizes of collections (see Sect. 8.4.1.3 Activity). The novel scoring items were hyperintensity on (fat-saturated) T1-weighted images and dominant feature of the tract (fibrous, granulation tissue, or pus). This resulted in good intrarater reliability, but the interrater reliability was not improved compared to the original Van Assche index. The modified van Assche index could be promising in the evaluation of therapy response because of the additional activity parameters but has yet to be studied for this purpose and potentially modified based on the responsiveness of the descriptors.

8.5.5 Differential Diagnosis

There are some considerations in the differential diagnosis of perianal Crohn's disease:

- Veins: It can be difficult to distinguish veins from fistulae because they both appear as hyperintense tubular structures on (fat-saturated) T2-weighted sequences and T1-weighted sequences. Distinctive factors are that most veins are symmetrical, tortuous, and thin-walled and are continuous with other veins. Tracts are often more straight and have a thicker wall, seen as a hypointense rim, and have an internal opening [32].
- Hemorrhoids and anal tags: Internal hemorrhoids can look like small subepithelial/submucosal abscesses on MRI, but when followed they originate in a vein. External hemorrhoids and anal tags are easily recognized at clinical examination [33].
- Pilonidal sinus: When a posterior track extends to the skin overlying the sacrum and gluteal region, it can be difficult to differentiate between a perianal fistula and a pilonidal sinus. The absence of intersphincteric involvement and absence of an internal opening distinguish pilonidal sinus from perianal fistula [34] (Fig. 8.14).
- Hidradenitis suppurativa extending to the anal sphincter region can be difficult to distinguish from an extensive fistula complex. Differences are less fistulae, less frequently sphincter involvement, more frequent granulomas, absence of rectal wall thickening, and bilateral disease in hidradenitis suppurativa [35] (Fig. 8.15).
- Tumor: In long-standing disease, cancer can develop within a track. It is therefore important to scrutinize the complete fistula for soft tissue not representing fibrous tissue or active track (Fig. 8.16).

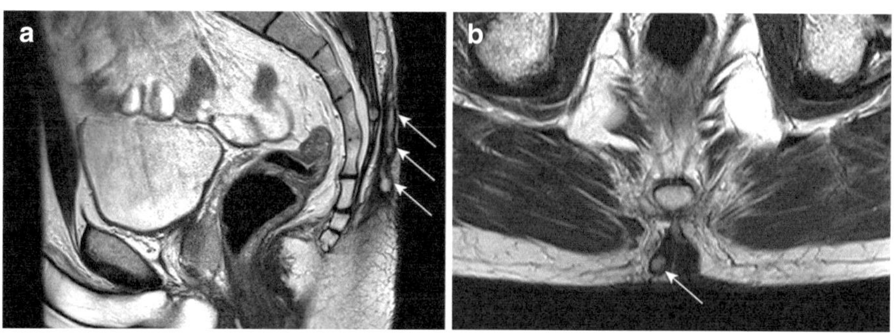

Fig. 8.14 Typical location of pilonidal sinus (arrows) at a sagittal T2-weighted sequence (**a**) and oblique axial T2-weighted sequence (**b**)

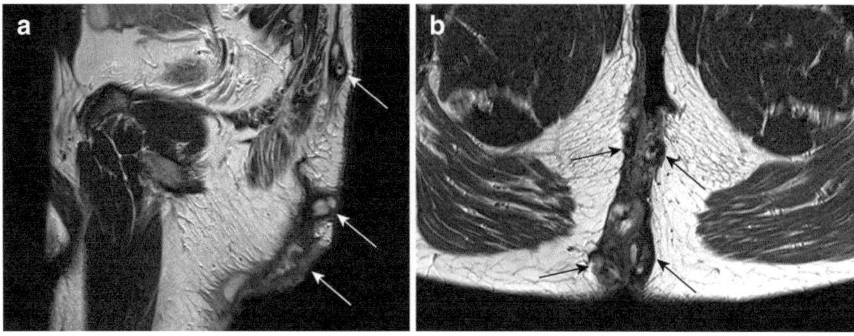

Fig. 8.15 Extensive fistulas (*arrows*) on a sagittal T2-weighted sequence (**a**) and oblique axial T2-weighted sequence (**b**) in a patient with Crohn's disease for which differential diagnoses hidradenitis suppurativa and pilonidal sinus were considered. A firm distinction could not be made based on these images, but due to history and extensiveness, fistulizing Crohn's disease was most likely

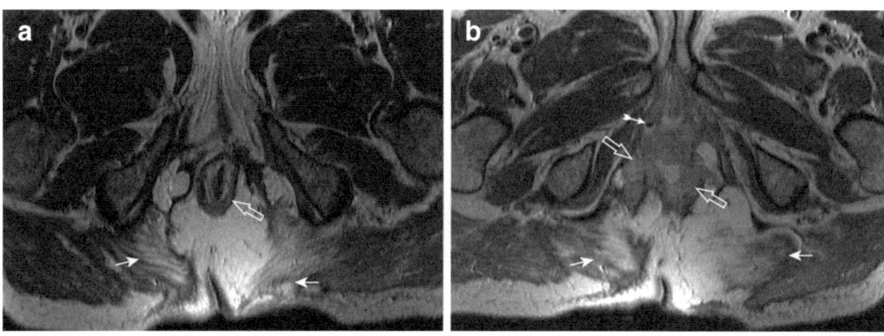

Fig. 8.16 Oblique axial T2-weighted images with 5 years between image **a** and **b** of a patient with extensive perianal Crohn's disease illustrating the development of a soft tissue mass at the anorectal canal (**b**) (*open arrows*) that was diagnosed as a malignant tumor. The short arrows indicate inflammation in the soft tissue and the tailed arrow an air configuration within a track

8.5.6 Structured Report

There are several possibilities of a structured evaluation of MRI for perianal Crohn's disease. Whichever approach chosen, there are key elements that need to be assessed and reported. It is important that the report is not merely a list of imaging findings but that the questions of the referring gastroenterologist or surgeon are addressed in a structured manner that will facilitate applying the imaging findings to patient management. The radiologist is very much helped in this by an informative referral by the gastroenterologist or surgeon with clear questions. Discussion with your gastroenterologists and surgeons to find the best way to clearly communicate the clinical questions and the MRI findings is important. Also, the pelvic anatomy is not always interpreted uniformly; discussion between radiologists and clinicians is crucial for adequate interpretation of anatomical location and to prevent miscommunication. Below is an example of a structured report; text between brackets should be replaced with the correct information.

General

Pelvic MRI according to perianal fistula protocol:

[***Specify performed sequences, directions, and contrast administration including agent and volume.***]

No imaging to compare with/comparison with [***imaging modality***] *from* [***date***]

Fistula*

[*New/known*] [*transsphincteric/intersphincteric/suprasphincteric/extrasphincteric/submucosal*] fistula tract [*left/right*] with [*supralevatoric/infralevatoric/other*] extension

Internal opening [*quadrant or clockwise location*] at [...] mm cranially from the lowest border of the sphincter complex**

Predominantly [*active/inactive]* fistula tract, consisting of [*granulation tissue/fluid/fibrous tissue*]

Other findings consist of [e.g., *setons, infiltration].*

Other perianal complications

No abscess or infiltrate/infiltrate at [*location*]/abscess at [*location*] with diameter of [... *x* ...] mm, filled with [*granulation tissue/fluid*]; no surrounding infiltrate/surrounding infiltrate

No proctitis/[*mild/severe*] proctitis with signs of [*mural thickening/infiltration/ulcerations/lymphadenopathy*]

No other perianal findings/other perianal findings are *[*e.g., *internal sphincter defect].*

Additional findings

No other relevant findings/other findings consist of [e.g., *free fluid, lymphadenopathy, uterus*, *or bone pathology*].

Conclusion

Answer the clinical questions, and report other relevant findings, preferably with bullet points.

(In case of clinical important findings necessitating immediate management, directly contact the referring physician or his/her replacement, and document this.)

*In case of several tracts defined by separate internal openings, repeat this paragraph for every tract.

** The distance to the anorectal junction can be added when this is close to the anorectal junction or if this is preferable for the clinician.

8.6 Conclusion

In conclusion, MRI has a pivotal role in the assessment of perianal Crohn's disease. Advantages compared to other imaging modalities are the ability to assess the entire pelvic region for extensive fistula tracts, intrinsic contrast resolution, and noninvasiveness. Using a phased-array surface coil, T2-weighted sequences and a T2-weighted sequence with fat suppression should be performed to adequately assess the perianal anatomy and fistula tracts. Additionally, it is recommended to perform a T1-weighted sequence with intravenous contrast agent to assess activity. The evaluation of perianal fistula on MRI should include a description of the anatomical location of a fistula in relation to the sphincter complex, internal opening, activity, presence of abscesses and proctitis, and response to therapy. Different classification systems, including activity parameters, have been developed for the assessment of therapeutic response but have not been validated fully. The evaluation and report of perianal Crohn's disease on MRI should have the purpose of aiding decisions regarding therapeutic strategy for the clinician, including guidance for possible surgical interventions.

References

1. Schwartz DA, Loftus EV, Tremaine WJ, Panaccione R, Harmsen WS, Zinsmeister AR, et al. The natural history of fistulizing Crohn's disease in Olmsted County, Minnesota. Gastroenterology. 2002;122:875–80. https://doi.org/10.1053/gast.2002.32362.
2. Eglinton TW, Barclay ML, Gearry RB, Frizelle FA. The spectrum of perianal Crohn's disease in a population-based cohort. Dis Colon Rectum. 2012;55:773–7. https://doi.org/10.1097/DCR.0b013e31825228b0.
3. Gecse KB, Bemelman W, Kamm MA, Stoker J, Khanna R, Ng SC, et al. A global consensus on the classification, diagnosis and multidisciplinary treatment of perianal fistulising Crohn's disease. Gut. 2014;63:1381–92. https://doi.org/10.1136/gutjnl-2013-306709.
4. Panes J, Bouhnik Y, Reinisch W, Stoker J, Taylor SA, Baumgart DC, et al. Imaging techniques for assessment of inflammatory bowel disease: joint ECCO and ESGAR evidence-based consensus guidelines. J Crohns Colitis. 2013;7:556–85. https://doi.org/10.1016/j.crohns.2013.02.020.
5. Kim DH, Carucci LR, Baker ME, Cash BD, Dillman JR, Feig BW, et al. ACR appropriateness criteria Crohn disease. J Am Coll Radiol. 2015;12:1048–1057.e4. https://doi.org/10.1016/j.jacr.2015.07.005.
6. Maaser C, Sturm M, Vavricka SR, Kucharzik T, Fiorino G, Annese V, et al. ECCO-ESGAR Guideline for Diagnostic Assessment in IBD Part 1: Initial diagnosis, monitoring of known IBD, detections of complications. J Crohns Colitis. 2018 (in press). https://doi.org/10.1093/ecco-jcc/jjy113.
7. Schwartz DA, Wiersema MJ, Dudiak KM, Fletcher JG, Clain JE, Tremaine WJ, et al. A comparison of endoscopic ultrasound, magnetic resonance imaging, and exam under anesthesia for evaluation of Crohn's perianal fistulas. Gastroenterology. 2001;121:1064–72. https://doi.org/10.1053/gast.2001.28676.
8. Buchanan GN, Halligan S, Bartram CI, Williams AB, Tarroni D, Cohen CRG. Clinical examination, endosonography, and MR imaging in preoperative assessment of fistula in ano: comparison with outcome-based reference standard. Radiology. 2004;233:674–81. https://doi.org/10.1148/radiol.2333031724.

9. Siddiqui MRS, Ashrafian H, Tozer P, Daulatzai N, Burling D, Hart A, et al. A diagnostic accuracy meta-analysis of endoanal ultrasound and MRI for perianal fistula assessment. Dis Colon Rectum. 2012;55:576–85. https://doi.org/10.1097/DCR.0b013e318249d26c.
10. Maconi G, Tonolini M, Monteleone M, Bezzio C, Furfaro F, Villa C, et al. Transperineal perineal ultrasound versus magnetic resonance imaging in the assessment of perianal Crohn's disease. Inflamm Bowel Dis. 2013;19:2737–43. https://doi.org/10.1097/01.MIB.0000436274.95722.e5.
11. Parks AG. Pathogenesis and treatment of fistula-in-ano. Br Med J. 1961;1:463–9.
12. Hughes LE. Surgical pathology and management of anorectal Crohn's disease. J R Soc Med. 1978;71:644–51. https://doi.org/10.1177/014107687807100904.
13. Halligan S, Stoker J. Imaging of fistula in ano. Radiology. 2006;239:18–33. https://doi.org/10.1148/radiol.2391041043.
14. Horsthuis K, Stoker J. MRI of perianal Crohn's disease. Am J Roentgenol. 2004;183:1309–15.
15. Dwarkasing S, Hussain SM, Hop WCJ, Krestin GP. Anovaginal fistulas: evaluation with endoanal MR imaging. Radiology. 2004;231:123–8. https://doi.org/10.1148/radiol.2311021190.
16. Sturm A, Maaser C, Calabrese E, Annese V, Fiorino G, Kucharzik T, et al. ECCO-ESGAR Guideline for Diagnostic Assessment in IBD Part 2: IBD scores and general principles and technical aspects. J Crohns Colitis. 2018 (in press). https://doi.org/10.1093/ecco-jcc/jjy114.
17. Dohan A, Eveno C, Oprea R, Pautrat K, Placé V, Pocard M, et al. Diffusion-weighted MR imaging for the diagnosis of abscess complicating fistula-in-ano: preliminary experience. Eur Radiol. 2014;24:2906–15. https://doi.org/10.1007/s00330-014-3302-y.
18. Hori M, Oto A, Orrin S, Suzuki K, Baron RL. Diffusion-weighted MRI: a new tool for the diagnosis of fistula in ano. J Magn Reson Imaging. 2009;30:1021–6. https://doi.org/10.1002/jmri.21934.
19. Horsthuis K, Lavini C, Bipat S, Stokkers P, Stoker J. Perianal Crohn disease: evaluation of dynamic contrast-enhanced MR imaging as an indicator of disease activity. Radiology. 2009;251:380–7. https://doi.org/10.1148/radiol.2512072128.
20. Ziech MLW, Lavini C, Bipat S, Ponsioen CY, Spijkerboer AM, Stokkers PCF, et al. Dynamic contrast-enhanced MRI in determining disease activity in perianal fistulizing Crohn disease: a pilot study. Am J Roentgenol. 2013;200:170–7. https://doi.org/10.2214/AJR.11.8276.
21. Pinson C, Dolores M, Cruypeninck Y, Koning E, Dacher JN, Savoye G, et al. Magnetization transfer ratio for the assessment of perianal fistula activity in Crohn's disease. Eur Radiol. 2017;27:80–7. https://doi.org/10.1007/s00330-016-4350-2.
22. Parks AG, Gordon PH, Hardcastle JD. A classification of fistula-in-ano. Br J Surg. 1976;63:1–12.
23. Samaan MA, Puylaert CAJ, Levesque BG, Zou GY, Stitt L, Taylor SA, et al. The development of a magnetic resonance imaging index for fistulising Crohn's disease. Aliment Pharmacol Ther. 2017;46:516–28. https://doi.org/10.1111/apt.14190.
24. Sandborn WJ, Fazio VW, Feagan BG, Hanauer SB. American Gastroenterological Association technical review on perianal Crohn's disease. Gastroenterology. 2003;125:1508–30. https://doi.org/10.1053/S0016-5085(03)01367-2.
25. Morris J, Spencer JA, Ambrose NS. MR imaging classification of perianal fistulas and its implications for patient management. Radiographics. 2000;20:623–35. https://doi.org/10.1148/radiographics.20.3.g00mc15623.
26. Van Assche G, Vanbeckevoort D, Bielen D, Coremans G, Aerden I, Noman M, et al. Magnetic resonance imaging of the effects of infliximab on perianal fistulizing Crohn's disease. Am J Gastroenterol. 2003;98:332–9. https://doi.org/10.1016/S0002-9270(02)05909-9.
27. Rociu E, Stoker J, Eijkemans MJ, Laméris JS. Normal anal sphincter anatomy and age- and sex-related variations at high-spatial-resolution endoanal MR imaging. Radiology. 2000;217:395–401. https://doi.org/10.1148/radiology.217.2.r00nv13395.
28. Tutein Nolthenius CJ, Bipat S, Mearadji B, Spijkerboer AM, Ponsioen CY, Montauban van Swijndregt AD, et al. MRI characteristics of proctitis in Crohn's disease on perianal MRI. Abdom Radiol. 2016;41:1918–30. https://doi.org/10.1007/s00261-016-0802-z.

29. Ng SC, Plamondon S, Gupta A, Burling D, Swatton A, Vaizey CJ, et al. Prospective evaluation of anti-tumor necrosis factor therapy guided by magnetic resonance imaging for Crohn's perineal fistulas. Am J Gastroenterol. 2009;104:2973–86. https://doi.org/10.1038/ajg.2009.509.
30. Karmiris K, Bielen D, Vanbeckevoort D, Vermeire S, Coremans G, Rutgeerts P, et al. Long-term monitoring of infliximab therapy for perianal fistulizing Crohn's disease by using magnetic resonance imaging. Clin Gastroenterol Hepatol. 2011;9:130–136.e1. https://doi.org/10.1016/j.cgh.2010.10.022.
31. Horsthuis K, Ziech MLW, Bipat S, Spijkerboer AM, de Bruine-Dobben AC, Hommes DW, et al. Evaluation of an MRI-based score of disease activity in perianal fistulizing Crohn's disease. Clin Imaging. 2011;35:360–5. https://doi.org/10.1016/j.clinimag.2010.09.003.
32. Stoker J, Rociu E, Zwamborn AW, Schouten WR, Laméris JS. Endoluminal MR imaging of the rectum and anus: technique, applications, and pitfalls. Radiographics. 1999;19:383–98. https://doi.org/10.1148/radiographics.19.2.g99mr01383.
33. Horsthuis K, Bipat S, Stokkers PCF, Stoker J. Magnetic resonance imaging for evaluation of disease activity in Crohn's disease: a systematic review. Eur Radiol. 2009;19:1450–60. https://doi.org/10.1007/s00330-008-1287-0.
34. Taylor SA, Halligan S, Bartram CI. Pilonidal sinus disease: MR imaging distinction from fistula in ano. Radiology. 2003;226:662–7. https://doi.org/10.1148/radiol.2263011758.
35. Monnier L, Dohan A, Amara N, Zagdanski AM, Drame M, Soyer P, et al. Anoperineal disease in Hidradenitis Suppurativa: MR imaging distinction from perianal Crohn's disease. Eur Radiol. 2017;27:4100–9. https://doi.org/10.1007/s00330-017-4776-1.

Cross-Sectional Imaging Indexes for Crohn's Disease

9

Jordi Rimola

Abstract

Objective assessment of disease activity and complications in Crohn's disease (CD) is critical to ensure accurate diagnosis and assessment of therapeutic response in both clinical practice and research. For recent clinical trials, patient selection and trial endpoints have been based on clinical symptoms and mucosal inflammation of the terminal ileum and large bowel determined on ileocolonoscopy. However, cross-sectional imaging methods have definite advantages over ileocolonoscopy and are potentially superior for use in CD clinical practice and trials. The development and validation of objective indexes of activity based on cross-sectional imaging will improve patient selection and assessment of the efficacy of new treatments.

9.1 Introduction

In Crohn's disease (CD), clinical decisions and new drug evaluation are based mainly on symptom control. Clinicians order changes to treatment to better manage symptoms associated with inflammatory activity (e.g., diarrhea, abdominal pain), impairment of general well-being, or extraintestinal manifestations. The Crohn's disease activity index (CDAI), based on the assessment of signs and symptoms plus measurement of hematocrit [1], has become the gold standard for assessing drug efficacy and the most important FDA-approvable endpoint for developing treatments for CD.

J. Rimola (✉)
Department of Radiology, Hospital Clínic of Barcelona, CIBEREHD, University of Barcelona, Barcelona, Spain
e-mail: jrimola@clinic.cat

J. Rimola (ed.), *Cross-Sectional Imaging in Crohn's Disease*,
https://doi.org/10.1007/978-3-319-96586-4_9

However, the CDAI, a composite score taking into account self-reported signs and symptoms of CD, correlates poorly with mucosal disease activity and has a high placebo rate. An analysis of data from the SONIC study showed that 18% of patients classified by the CDAI as having moderate-to-severe disease (CDAI > 220) had no ulcers at endoscopy [2]. Moreover, after therapeutic intervention, 47% of patients who were classified as in remission by the CDAI (CDAI < 150) still had ulcers, and 35% of those whose mucosa had healed were classified as still having active disease. On the other hand, patients with CD under sustained clinical remission may still suffer from ulcerative lesions [3], which have been linked to increased need for surgical resections [4].

Given the mismatch between patient-reported symptoms and signs of disease and evidence of mucosal inflammation, the FDA currently holds that the primary endpoints in clinical trials to support approval of novel molecules with indication for CD should include ileocolonoscopy (ILC) findings as well as symptoms and signs (specifically abdominal pain and stool frequency).

The gold standard for assessing lesions in CD is ILC, but it has inherent limitations [5]. It requires intense bowel cleansing and is cumbersome, so many patients with symptomatic CD may complain to undergo the examination. Importantly, complete assessment is not always possible; in patients with active CD, the right colon can be reached in 90% of examinations, but the terminal ileum in only 75% [6]. Finally, like clinical assessment, ILC has a low sensitivity for the detection of penetrating complications [7–9] (intraabdominal fistulas and abscesses), which are usually exclusion criteria for clinical trials, given the risk of immunosuppressive therapies worsening the septic component of these lesions.

Recent evidence indicates that cross-sectional imaging techniques are reliable alternatives to ILC. Not only are they accurate in the assessment of mucosal lesions, they also offer some advantages, such as enabling the assessment of extramural complications (e.g., fistulas and abscesses) and determining the functional repercussions of stenotic lesions [7, 10].

This chapter discusses cross-sectional imaging-based indexes for the objective detection of disease activity and characterization of disease severity in CD, providing practical recommendations for the optimal use of these scores for luminal and perianal disease in clinical practice and research.

9.2 Indexes for Small and Colon Activity Assessment

9.2.1 Selecting the Appropriate Indexes

Some of cross-sectional indexes are constructed by selection of parameters that are associated with the presence of disease activity and/or are indicators of the presence of severe disease based on overall radiologist assessment [11–17]. The number of parameters present defines the existence of active disease and level of severity, usually limited to three-point or four-point global scale (i.e., inactive, mild, moderate, or severe). Using this model, the lack of strict criteria in selecting the variables that compose these indexes contributes to the heterogeneity of the parameters included in each index.

By contrast, the derivation of indexes based on regression models that predict activity assessed by a valid external gold standard (histology or endoscopy) is more stringent since only the variables with independent predictor value for severity and activity are selected, whereas those without a proven independent predictor value are excluded from the scoring system, optimizing the evaluation of the imaging technique. The downside of using indexes based on regression models is that the derived indexes may not be easily applicable in clinical practice if they entail the quantitative measurement of too many or too difficult descriptors or are based in complex formulas. Therefore, these limitations may be overcome by the simplification of indexes in terms of data capture and calculation, without compromising their overall accuracy.

9.2.2 Cross-Sectional Index for Luminal Crohn's Disease

There are no formal indexes on luminal activity based on ultrasonography or computed tomography enterography (CTE). However, in the field of CTE, the EMBARK study developed a combined ileocolonoscopy-CTE score, applied in a subgroup of CD patients who underwent both investigative procedures. Data on severity could be obtained by using either endoscopy or CTE, so that the incorporation of both ILC and CTE into a single measure increased biomarker performance in CD (Table 9.1) [18].

Among different MRE-based indexes published in the literature, only few of them had been derived using valid external reference standard (i.e., endoscopy or histology) and using descriptors identified in multivariate analysis as independent predictors for detecting activity and severity.

The *magnetic resonance index of activity* (MaRIA) is the best-characterized MRE-based index of activity. The MaRIA index is a composite score that takes into account bowel wall thickness (in millimeters), MR image signal enhancement by gadolinium-based intravascular contrast agent, and observation of ulceration and

Table 9.1 Definitions used to assign combined scores incorporating findings from either ileocolonoscopy or CT enterography on EMBARK study

Score	Disease severity	Length of active region
0	• None	None
1	• Aphthous erosion • Hyperenhancement with no or equivocal wall thickening (3–5 mm)	<50% of bowel segment
2	• Large ulcers • ≥5 mm wall thickening (at thickest region) with hyperenhancement	50–75% of bowel segment
3	• Very large ulcers • ≥5 mm with wall thickening, hyperenhancement and perienteric fat stranding, ulcers, or wall thickening >10 mm	>75% of bowel segment

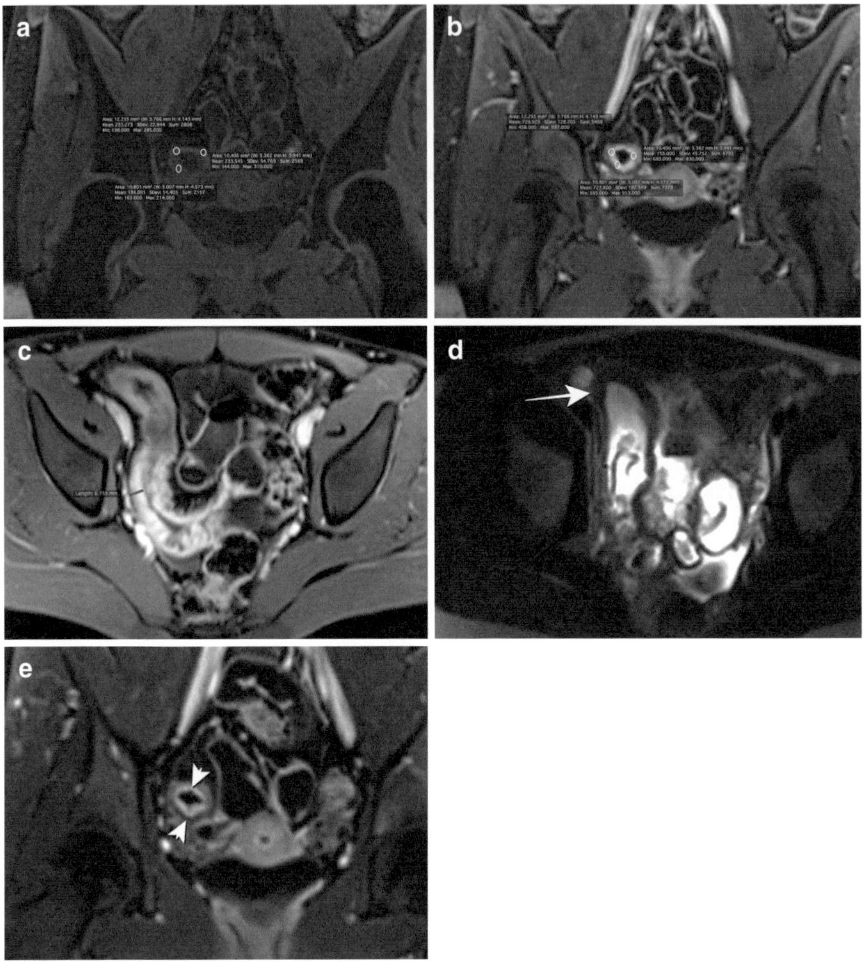

Fig. 9.1 The MaRIA index grades disease activity using relative contrast enhancement (ROIs in **a** and **b**), by measuring wall thickness (line in **c**) and identifying the presence of edema (**d**, *arrow*) and ulcerations (**e**, *arrowheads*). Both edema and ulcerations were present in this ileal segment (*arrows* in **d** and **e** respectively). For scoring of the London index, wall thickness (**c**) and mural T2 signal (**d**) are assessed to calculate an acute inflammation score (AIS). In this patient, there is a moderate increase in mural T2 signal (**d**, *arrow*)

edema (hyperintensity on T2-weighted sequences) (Fig. 9.1). The sub-score at segmental level is calculated for five colonic segments (rectum, sigmoid colon, descending colon, transverse colon, and ascending colon) plus for the terminal ileum. MaRIA was derived as a simplified score to quantify disease activity from MRI findings in each segment:

$$\begin{aligned}\text{MaRIAseg} = {} & \left(1.5 \times \text{Wall thickness}\right) + \left(0.02 \times \text{relative contrast enhancement}\right) \\ & + \left(5 \times \text{edema}\right) + \left(10 \times \text{ulcers at MRE}\right)\end{aligned}$$

where WT means bowel wall thickness in mm measured at the thickest point in the segment; edema and ulcer are each assigned a value of 1 when there is evidence of either in the segment (or 0 when not). RCE represents the relative contrast enhancement between pre- and post-gadolinium T1 and can be calculated as follows: RCE=((WSI postgadolinium–WSI pregadolinium)/(WSI pregadolinium))×100 × (SD noise pregadolinium/SD noise postgadolinium), where SD noise pregadolinium corresponds to the average of three SDs of the signal intensity measured outside of the body before gadolinium injection, and SD noise postgadolinium corresponds to the SD of the same noise after gadolinium administration.

The global MaRIA score is computed as the sum total of the sub-scores.

In order to categorize the severity of each individual segment evaluated by MRE, two different cutoffs were defined. A MaRIA sub-score of ≥7 is indicative of bowel segments with active CD, and a sub-score of ≥11 units identifies segments with moderate-to-severe CD activity, with ulcers at endoscopy.

The MaRIA score was devised to be highly accurate in detecting active disease or even better for the detection of severe inflammation when compared with an objective endoscopic score, the Crohn's Disease Endoscopic Index of Severity (CDEIS), a widely used, objective endoscopic score [19, 20]. MaRIA score was used to determine the responsiveness of MRE after induction treatment in CD patients following medical therapeutic intervention showing high accuracy for detecting mucosal healing (accuracy 0.83 for a cuttof $MaRIA_{seg} < 7$) at segmental level (Table 9.2) and at patient level (accuracy 0.86 for a cutoff $MaRIA_{global} < 50$) [21]. Contrary to the work of Ordás et al. [21], Stoppino et al. [22] reported on observations of "global MaRIA" change in response to anti-TNF at week 26 and suggest that the optimal cutoff point for identification of patients that had achieved mucosal healing at week 26 is 30.8. It is important to highlight that in contrast to $MaRIA_{global}$ including six segments, in the work of Stoppino et al. [22] is scored as the summation of $MaRIA_{seg}$ across only five segments.

Similarities between segment scores for colon segments and proximal and distal small bowel segments have been reported. Takenaka et al. [23] have reported that using $MaRIA_{seg}$ cutoffs of <7 and ≥11 is as accurate at predicting double-balloon enteroscopy appearance of the mucosa in the jejunum and proximal and terminal ileum than in the colon. Furthermore, these authors have also reported that $MaRIA_{seg}$ is highly correlated with the endoscopic score SES-CD.

Table 9.2 Diagnostic accuracy of MaRIA at segment level derived from the derivation and validation cohort for assessment of disease activity and severity

	MaRIA				
	AUC	R^2	Cutoff	Sens	Spec
Active disease	0.93	0.72	≥7	0.87	0.87
Severe disease	0.97	0.71	≥11	0.92	0.92
Mucosal healing	0.83	0.51	<7	0.85	0.78

Derived in [19] and [21]
AUC receiver operating characteristic area under the curve, *Sens* sensitivity, *Spec* specificity
Ileocolonoscopy was the reference standard.

However, some drawbacks of the MaRIA index have to be acknowledged. The main limitation as far as the assessment of therapeutic response is concerned is that normal segments contribute to the overall MaRIA score, while in patients with surgically resected segments an underestimation of the global score occurs. With regard to the easiness for its calculation, although it only takes into account four items, its computation can be cumbersome and time consuming because two variables are quantitative (thickening, contrast enhancement) and must be calculated in all colonic segments and in the terminal ileum.

The *acute inflammation score* (AIS) is another MRE index and is composite of two descriptors (mural thickness and mural T2 signal) that are computed in a semi-quantitative fashion using a four-point scale. It was originally derived for scoring the inflammation on the terminal ileum using histopathology as gold standard:

$$\text{AIS} = 1.79 + (1.34 \times \text{mural thickness}) + (0.94 \times \text{mural T2 score})$$

An AIS of 4.1 was determined as the best cutoff to define presence of active disease with an AUC of 0.77 and demonstrated a moderate degree of correlation with inflammation at histopathology (Kendall's tau = 0.40) [24].

The same group derived an extended version of AIS to include simply the sum of all MRI parameters which had an individual strength of association of at least $p < 0.1$ in the derivation analysis including mural thickness, mural T2 signal, perimural T2 signal, and contrast enhancement. However, its addition to the original index marginally improved the correlation with the AIS score.

In addition to its accuracy, the main advantage over other indexes is that AIS can be calculated faster. However, the lack of defined cutoff point to define the presence of severe inflammation (ulceration) that can be used as inclusion criteria in clinical trials and lack of data about responsiveness of this index after medical interventions are the main limitations of this index to be used in clinical trials.

The *Nancy score* was the first one to include diffusion-weighted imaging (DWI) sequence as independent predictor of active disease [25]. Its derivation was based on the presence of inflammatory lesions at endoscopic colonic evaluation including erythema, edema, pseudopolyps, aphthoid ulcers, and ulceration. Nancy index includes six descriptors at MRI: DWI hyperintensity, rapid gadolinium enhancement after intravenous contrast medium administration, differentiation between the mucosa-submucosa complex and the muscularis propria, bowel wall thickening (>5 mm), mural edema, and the presence of ulceration, although only the presence of DWI hyperintensity and increased bowel wall thickening were independent predictor of the presence of endoscopic inflammation. The presence and absence of each descriptor in a given segment is rated in a binary way ("1" when present and "0" when absent). The segmental Nancy MR score is calculated as the sum of the numerical values obtained among the six descriptors for a given segment. The total Nancy MR was calculated as the sum of each segmental score in a patient, with values ranging from 0 to 36. A MR-score-S >2 detected endoscopic inflammation in the colon with a sensitivity and specificity of 58.33% and 84.48%, respectively, with an AUROC of 0.779 ($p = 0.0001$). The correlation between segmental index and SES-CD was moderate ($r = 0.54$).

This index was not further validated in a prospective cohort neither tested for assessing therapeutic response to medical intervention.

Finally, a novel index, very similar to MaRIA index but using diffusion-weighted imaging (DWI) sequence instead of contrast enhancement, had been recently developed, called *DWI-MaRIA* score or *Clermont score* [26]. To derive and validate DWI-MaRIA score, the same MRE (MaRIA) was considered the reference standard. Not strangely, wall thickness, mural edema, and ulcerations were included as independent predictors for activity, together with the apparent coefficient of diffusion (ADC), using $\text{MaRIA}_{\text{seg}}$ as dependent variable. Clermont score was derived to quantify disease activity from MRI findings in each segment as follows:

$$\begin{aligned}\text{Clermont}_{\text{seg}} = &\left(1.646 \times \text{Wall thickness}\right) + \left(-1.321 \times \text{ADC}\right) \\ &+ \left(5.613 \times \text{edema}\right) + \left(8.306 \times \text{ulcers at MRE}\right) + 5.039\end{aligned}$$

A Clermont sub-score of ≥8.4 is indicative of bowel segments with active CD, and a sub-score of ≥12.5 units identifies segments with moderate-to-severe CD activity, with ulcers at endoscopy. As expected, a very close correlation had been found between both MaRIA and Clermont indexes [26], being almost perfect ($r = 0.99$) in the terminal ileum but lower in the colon.

The responsiveness of Clermont index after induction treatment in CD patients following medical therapeutic intervention showed a good specificity (76.5%), whereas the sensitivity was only 60% for endoscopic mucosal healing at segment level [27].

The Clermont score had emerged as a promising biomarker of bowel inflammation in CD, especially useful when gadolinium cannot be given. However, confirmatory studies are currently lacking [28]. The main limitation for the applicability of this index is the current lack of standardized method for DWI acquisition including technical aspects and bowel preparation that may affect the accuracy of this index when different parameters were used to set up DWI sequence [29].

9.2.3 Reproducibility of the Indexes

Different comparative studies of these two indexes using ILC indexes as reference standard validated both indexes [29, 30].

Reproducibility of these indexes is a critical step to be considered useful evaluative instruments. Specifically, moderate-to-good degrees of interobserver agreement (0.42–0.69) among expert readers had been detected for each MR descriptors of both MaRIA and AIS indexes in the colonic and terminal ileum segments [30]. Another pilot study including 19 CD patients, both test–retest and inter-reader reliability for segmental MaRIA score in the terminal ileum were excellent with correlation coefficients ranging from 0.92 to 0.97. However, reader agreement was lower in the proximal small bowel segments (0.59 and 0.72), and the strength of correlation of the MaRIA score with CDEIS was lower than in the original single-site validation study ($r = 0.63$; $p < 0.01$), as expected with central read multisite dissemination.

9.3 Indexes for Perianal Disease

Although various clinical scoring systems for assessing perianal disease have been developed, few scoring systems are based on or include pelvic MRI findings. Various authors consider pelvic MRI the gold standard imaging modality for detecting and characterizing abscesses and fistulas [31]. Scoring systems should enable assessment of the severity of disease and of the response to treatment. The lack of a validated outcome measure has constrained research in this field.

In clinical practice, the most widely accepted approach for the initial assessment of perianal disease consists of physical examination of the perianal area (mainly the number of draining external openings) and pelvic MRI examination including anatomical description of the existing fistula tracks and the parameters of inflammation. In follow-up, the correlation between fistula healing and favorable clinical course is well accepted, and perianal disease is normally monitored by clinical evaluation (decrease from baseline in number of open draining fistulas) [32]. However, because there is no consensus about the optimal time to reassess perianal disease to determine whether fistulas have completely healed, regular pelvic MRI follow-up does not form part of the standard of care in most institutions, and MRI reassessment is limited to patients with unfavorable clinical outcome.

Nevertheless, in research, pelvic MRI is an essential element in patient follow-up in clinical trials of novel drugs. Even in this scenario, however, despite MRI's unquestionable value in characterizing fistula anatomy, the most appropriate MRI methods and criteria for complete fistula healing have yet to be established [33, 34].

MRI-based scores provide a more objective measure of fistula activity than simple clinical evaluation, as the simple closure of external openings does not ensure deep fistula healing or the absence of complications [31, 32].

9.3.1 The Van Assche Index

The Van Assche Index (VAI) was originally developed to fill the need for a standardized tool that could measure the response of perianal fistulizing CD to medical therapy [35], thus obviating the need for each patient to serve as his or her own control to determine whether perianal disease improved or worsened [36]. The VAI score rates the severity of the perianal fistulizing process based on the MRI findings, including the number of fistula tracks, fistula location according to Parks classification, fistula extension, hyperintensity on T2-weighted images, collections (≥3 mm in diameter), and rectal wall involvement (Table 9.3). Based primarily on radiological expertise, some of the descriptors used in the VAI have been criticized. For

Table 9.3 The Van Assche index, MRI-based score for severity of perianal Crohn's disease

Descriptor	Categories	Scoring
Number of fistula tracts	• None • Single, unbranched • Single, branched • Multiple	0 1 2 3
Location	• Extrasphincteric or intersphincteric • Trans-sphincteric • Suprasphincteric	1 2 3
Extension	• Infralevatoric • Supralevatoric	1 2
Hyperintensity on T2-weighted images	• Absent • Mild • Pronounced	0 4 8
Collections (cavities >3 mm diameter)	• Absent • Present	0 4
Rectal wall involvement	• Normal • Thickened	0 2

instance, the proposed 3 mm cutoff for the diameter of fluid collections is not useful for guiding clinical decisions, because many fistula tracts, especially in the context of complex fistulas, have a diameter greater than 3 mm, and these are considered fistulas, not abscesses. Moreover, the scoring system proposed for each descriptor (especially for extensions and anatomical classification of fistulas) is controversial, and some descriptors (e.g., anatomical location of the track) may not be responsive to treatment.

Nevertheless, changes in the VAI, especially T2 signal intensity of fistula tracts, correlate with clinical disease activity and with clinical response to immunosuppressant treatment on short-term follow-up [35, 37]. Savoye-Collet et al. [38] found that the VAI score (particularly T2 hyperintensity) significantly improved after 1 year of infliximab therapy. However, other studies found that the VAI was insensitive to change in patients with reduced fistula caliber during long-term follow-up [33, 39]. Finally, the lack of validated cutoff values associated with response or fistula healing hinders the use of this index as an endpoint in clinical trials [34, 38].

9.3.2 The Modified Van Assche Index (mVAI)

To overcome the aforementioned limitations of the VAI, a modified version was developed. In the derivation process, fistula descriptors were initially selected based on their intra- and inter-reader reliability, and a final index was generated using a visual analog scale for global assessment of severity as an outcome criterion [40]. The final modified version of VAI includes extension, hyperintensity on T2-weighted images, rectal wall involvement, inflammatory mass (incorporating the components of the descriptor "collections" in the original VAI as well as additional features),

Table 9.4 The modified Van Assche index, MRI-based score for severity of perianal Crohn's disease

Descriptor	Modified index	Item weight	Definition developed through initial consensus
Extension	• Absent	0	
	• Infralevatoric	1	Extends upward in the ischioanal fossa but remains below the levator ani muscle
	• Horseshoe configuration	2	Extends into the intersphincteric space on both sides of the midline
	• Supralevatoric	3	Extends upward in the intersphincteric plane and over the top of the levator ani muscle
Hyperintensity on T2-weighted images	• Absent	0	No hyperintensity visible, only scar tissue
	• Mild	1	Slight increase in signal intensity but less than nearby, in- plane vessels
	• Pronounced	2	Tract showing equal or greater signal hyperintensity than nearby in-plane vessels
Rectal wall involvement (proctitis)	• Absence	0	Normal appearance of rectal wall
	• Present	2	Increased wall thickness and size of mesorectal lymph nodes (>5 mm), creeping fat, increased perimural T2 signal, and enhancement
Inflammatory mass	• Absent	0	No inflammatory mass
	• Diffuse	1	Diffuse inflammation of surrounding tissues
	• Focal	2	Lesion >3 mm in diameter on T2-weighted images (but does not include linear tracts with diameter >3 mm) with diffuse enhancement on T1-weighted post-contrast images (i.e., granulation tissue)
	• Collection – small	3	Circumscribed cavity 3–10 mm in diameter (but does not include linear tracts with diameter >3 mm) Hyperintense appearance on fat-saturated T2-weighted images with rim enhancement on T1-weighted post-contrast images
	• Collection – medium	4	As defined above except diameter measures 11–20 mm
	• Collection – large	5	As defined above except diameter measures >20 mm
Dominant feature of primary tract and extensions	• Predominantly fibrous	0	>50% of tract has a fibrotic appearance (i.e., hypointense on fat-saturated T2-weighted images)
	• Predominantly filled with granulation tissue	1	>50% of tract is filled with granulation tissue (i.e., hyperintense on fat-saturated T2-weighted images with enhancement of contents and wall on T1-weighted post-contrast images)
	• Predominantly filled with fluid or pus	2	>50% of tract is filled with fluid or pus (i.e., hyperintense on fat-saturated T2-weighted images with no enhancement of contents on fat-saturated T1-weighted post-contrast images [though lining of tract may enhance])

and dominant feature of primary tract and extension (Table 9.4). Before it can be universally adopted, the mVAI's responsiveness must be tested by comparing baseline and posttreatment MRI findings in patients receiving a treatment of known efficacy, ideally in a randomized controlled trial.

9.4 Index for Bowel Damage: The Lémann Index

CD is a progressive disease, so it is important to determine the impact of therapeutic interventions on damage progression. This can be difficult because it requires separating the long-term effects of a treatment from its short-term effects on symptoms. For these reasons, an international initiative recently developed the Lémann index to determine the progression of CD over time, focusing on digestive tract damage rather than on the degree of inflammatory activity [41].

Designed to measure the cumulative bowel damage in all segments of the digestive tract, the Lémann index is based on resections and the extent and severity of stricturing and penetrating lesions on MRI and endoscopy.

To determine the factors associated with digestive damage progression, a French group tracked Lémann index scores and retrospectively reviewed magnetic resonance enterography findings in a cohort of 221 CD patients followed for 2–10 years. They found that high Lémann index scores at the first evaluation, time, persistent clinical activity, and past history of intestinal resection were associated with damage [42].

In a prospective study tracking the Lémann index in a cohort of CD patients receiving anti-TNF, Fiorino et al. [43] found that the index was sensitive to change, indicating that anti-TNFs were able to reverse damage in some patients. A Lémann index >4.8 identified subjects with bowel damage, and an increase in Lémann index >0.3 during the follow-up identified damage progression. Patients with progression of bowel damage were more likely to require major abdominal surgery.

Thus, despite the initial assumption that the Lémann index was likely to increase with the disease duration, the Lémann index as currently defined can also decrease over time. This seems reasonable, given that the part of this index related to stricturing lesions includes potentially reversible inflammatory components (e.g., wall thickening, contrast enhancement, stricture, and prestenotic dilation), and the part of the index related to penetrating lesions also includes potentially reversible components (e.g., ulcerations, fistulas and phlegmon/abscesses). Nevertheless, this study showed that progression in Lémann index is associated with worse outcomes, including subsequent need for surgery.

In a more recent study, the same group evaluated the prognostic value of disease activity and severity in early CD by the Lémann index and MaRIA score in 142 consecutive patients followed up for 4.9 years. Bowel damage and the Lémann score, but not severity as expressed by the MaRIA score, were independent prognostic factors for predicting intestinal surgery (HR: 3.21 and 1.11, respectively, $p < 0.001$) and CD-related hospitalization (HR: 1.88, $p = 0.002$, and 1.08, $p < 0.001$, respectively) [44].

9.5 Conclusion

Cross-sectional imaging methods have emerged as potentially superior to ILC in CD for clinical practice and research. The development and validation of indexes of activity and severity will allow their implementation as potential biomarkers for selecting patients and assessing treatment efficacy for both luminal and perianal disease. The Lémann index, by contrast, was designed to determine the evolution of bowel damage over time. As expected, this index was found to be reversible, suggesting that further improvements on the current version of the index are needed.

References

1. Best W, Becktel J, Singleton JW, Kern F Jr. Development of a Crohn's disease activity index. National Cooperative Crohn's Disease Study. Gastroenterology. 1976;70:439–44.
2. Peyrin-Biroulet L, Reinisch W, Colombel J-F, Mantzaris GJ, Kornbluth A, Diamond R, et al. Clinical disease activity, C-reactive protein normalisation and mucosal healing in Crohn's disease in the SONIC trial. Gut. 2014;63:88–95.
3. Lémann M, Mary JY, Colombel JF, Duclos B, Soule JC, Lerebours E, et al. A randomized, double-blind, controlled withdrawal trial in Crohn's disease patients in long-term remission on azathioprine. Gastroenterology. 2005;128:1812–8.
4. Allez M, Lemann M, Cattan P, Jian R, Modigliani R. Long term outcome of patients with active Crohn's disease exhibiting extensive and deep ulcerations at colonoscopy. Am J Gastroenterol. 2002;97:947–53.
5. Gomollón F, Dignass A, Annese V, Tilg H, Van Assche G, Lindsay JO, et al. 3rd European evidence-based consensus on the diagnosis and management of Crohn's disease 2016: part 1: diagnosis and medical management. J Crohns Colitis. 2017;11:3–25.
6. Jauregui-Amezaga A, Rimola J, Ordás I, Rodríguez S, Ramírez-Morros A, Gallego M, et al. Value of endoscopy and MRI for predicting intestinal surgery in patients with Crohn's disease in the era of biologics. Gut. 2015;64:1397–402.
7. Samuel S, Bruining DH, Loftus EV, Becker B, Fletcher JG, Mandrekar JN, et al. Endoscopic skipping of the distal terminal ileum in Crohn's disease can lead to negative results from ileocolonoscopy. Clin Gastroenterol Hepatol. 2012;10:1253–9.
8. Solem CA, Loftus EV, Fletcher JG, Baron TH, Gostout CJ, Petersen BT, et al. Small-bowel imaging in Crohn's disease: a prospective, blinded, 4-way comparison trial. Gastrointest Endosc. 2008;68:255–66.
9. García-Bosch O, Ordás I, Aceituno M, Rodríguez S, Ramírez AM, Gallego M, et al. Comparison of diagnostic accuracy and impact of MRI and colonoscopy for the management of Crohn's disease. J Crohns Colitis. 2016;10:663–9.
10. Siddiki HA, Fidler JL, Fletcher JG, Burton SS, Huprich JE, Hough DM, et al. Prospective comparison of state-of-the-art MR enterography and CT enterography in small-bowel Crohn's disease. AJR Am J Roentgenol. 2009;193:113–21.
11. Girometti R, Zuiani C, Toso F, Brondani G, Sorrentino D. MRI scoring system including dynamic motility evaluation in assessing the activity of Crohn's disease of the terminal ileum. Acad Radiol. 2008;15:153–64.
12. Sailer J, Peloschek P, Reinisch W, Vogelsang H, Turetschek K, Schima W. Anastomotic recurrence of Crohn's disease after ileocolic resection: comparison of MR enteroclysis with endoscopy. Eur Radiol. 2008;18:2512–21.

13. Hyun SB, Kitazume Y, Nagahori M, Toriihara A, Fujii T, Tsuchiya K, et al. Magnetic resonance enterocolonography is useful for simultaneous evaluation of small and large intestinal lesions in Crohn's disease. Inflamm Bowel Dis. 2011;17:1063–72.
14. Laghi A, Borrelli O, Paolantonio P, Dito L, Bueno de Mesquita M, Falconieri P, et al. Contrast enhanced magnetic resonance imaging of the terminal ileum in children with Crohn's disease. Gut. 2003;52:393–7.
15. Neye H, Voderholzer W, Rickes S, Weber J, Wermke W, Lochs H. Evaluation of criteria for the activity of Crohn's disease by power Doppler sonography. Dig Dis. 2004;22:67–72.
16. Drews B, Barth TFE, Hänle MM, Muche R, Pauls S, Klaus J, et al. Comparison of sonographically measured bowel wall vascularity, histology, and disease activity in Crohn's disease. Eur Radiol. 2009;19:1379–86.
17. Chiorean MV, Sandrasegaran K, Saxena R, Maglinte DD, Nakeeb A, Johnson CS. Correlation of CT enteroclysis with surgical pathology in Crohn's disease. Am J Gastroenterol. 2007;102:2541–50.
18. Faubion WA, Fletcher JG, Byrne SO, Feagan BG, De Villiers WJS, Salzberg B, et al. EMerging BiomARKers in Inflammatory Bowel Disease (EMBARK) study identifies fecal calprotectin, serum MMP9, and serum IL-22 as a novel combination of biomarkers for Crohn's disease activity: role of cross-sectional imaging. Am J Gastroenterol. 2013;108:1891–900.
19. Rimola J, Rodriguez S, Garcia-Bosch O, Ordas I, Ayala E, Aceituno M, et al. Magnetic resonance for assessment of disease activity and severity in ileocolonic Crohn's disease. Gut. 2009;58:1113–20.
20. Rimola J, Ordás I, Rodriguez S, García-Bosch O, Aceituno M, Llach J, et al. Magnetic resonance imaging for evaluation of Crohn's disease. Inflamm Bowel Dis. 2011;17:1759–68.
21. Ordás I, Rimola J, Rodríguez S, Paredes JM, Martínez-Pérez MJ, Blanc E, et al. Accuracy of magnetic resonance enterography in assessing response to therapy and mucosal healing in patients with Crohn's disease. Gastroenterology. 2014;146:374–82.
22. Stoppino LP, Della Valle N, Rizzi S, Cleopazzo E, Centola A, Iamele D, et al. Magnetic resonance enterography changes after antibody to tumor necrosis factor (anti-TNF) alpha therapy in Crohn's disease: correlation with SES-CD and clinical-biological markers. BMC Med Imaging. 2016;16:1–9.
23. Takenaka K, Ohtsuka K, Kitazume Y, Nagahori M, Fujii T, Saito E, et al. Correlation of the endoscopic and magnetic resonance scoring systems in the deep small intestine in Crohn's disease. Inflamm Bowel Dis. 2015;21:1832–8.
24. Steward MJ, Punwani S, Proctor I, Adjei-Gyamfi Y, Chatterjee F, Bloom S, et al. Non-perforating small bowel Crohn's disease assessed by MRI enterography: derivation and histopathological validation of an MR-based activity index. Eur J Radiol. 2012;81:2080–8.
25. Oussalah A, Laurent V, Bruot O, Bressenot A, Bigard M-A, Régent D, et al. Diffusion-weighted magnetic resonance without bowel preparation for detecting colonic inflammation in inflammatory bowel disease. Gut. 2010;59:1056–65.
26. Hordonneau C, Buisson A, Scanzi J, Goutorbe F, Pereira B, Borderon C, et al. Diffusion-weighted magnetic resonance imaging in ileocolonic Crohn's disease: validation of quantitative index of activity. Am J Gastroenterol. 2014;109:89–98.
27. Buisson A, Pereira B, Goutte M, Reymond M, Allimant C, Obritin-Guilhen H, et al. Magnetic resonance index of activity (MaRIA) and Clermont score are highly and equally effective MRI indices in detecting mucosal healing in Crohn's disease. Dig Liver Dis. 2017;49:1211–7.
28. Dohan A, Taylor S, Hoeffel C, Barret M, Allez M, Dautry R, et al. Diffusion-weighted MRI in Crohn's disease: current status and recommendations. J Magn Reson Imaging. 2016;44:1381–96.
29. Rimola J, Alvarez-Cofiño A, Pérez-Jeldres T, Ayuso C, Alfaro I, Rodríguez S, et al. Comparison of three magnetic resonance enterography indices for grading activity in Crohn's disease. J Gastroenterol. 2017;52:585–93.
30. Tielbeek JAW, Makanyanga JC, Bipat S, Pendsé DA, Nio CY, Vos FM, et al. Grading Crohn disease activity with MRI: interobserver variability of MRI features, MRI scoring of sever-

ity, and correlation with Crohn disease endoscopic index of severity. AJR Am J Roentgenol. 2013;201:1220–8.
31. Gecse KB, Bemelman W, Kamm MA, Stoker J, Khanna R, Ng SC, et al. A global consensus on the classification, diagnosis and multidisciplinary treatment of perianal fistulising Crohn's disease. Gut. 2014;63:1381–92.
32. Schwartz DA, Ghazi LJ, Regueiro M, Fichera A, Zoccali M, Ong EMW, et al. Guidelines for the multidisciplinary management of Crohn's perianal fistulas. Inflamm Bowel Dis. 2015;21:723–30.
33. Horsthuis K, Ziech MLW, Bipat S, Spijkerboer AM, de Bruine-Dobben AC, Hommes DW, et al. Evaluation of an MRI-based score of disease activity in perianal fistulizing Crohn's disease. Clin Imaging. 2011;35:360–5.
34. Tozer P, Ng SC, Siddiqui MR, Plamondon S, Burling D, Gupta A, et al. Long-term MRI-guided combined anti-TNF and thiopurine therapy for Crohn's perianal fistulas. Inflamm Bowel Dis. 2012;18:1825–34.
35. Van Assche G, Vanbeckevoort D, Bielen D, Coremans G, Aerden I, Noman M, et al. Magnetic resonance imaging of the effects of infliximab on perianal fistulizing Crohn's disease. Am J Gastroenterol. 2003;98:332–9.
36. Bell S, Williams A, Wiesel P, Wilkinson K, Cohen R, Kamm M. The clinical course of fistulating Crohn's disease. Aliment Pharmacol Ther. 2003;17:1145–51.
37. Horsthuis K, Lavini C, Bipat S, Stokkers PC, Stoker J. Perianal Crohn disease: evaluation of dynamic contrast-enhanced MR imaging as an indicator of disease activity. Radiology. 2009;251:380–7.
38. Savoye-Collet C, Savoye G, Koning E, Dacher JN, Lerebours E. Fistulizing perianal Crohn's disease: contrast-enhanced magnetic resonance imaging assessment at 1 year on maintenance anti-TNF-alpha therapy. Inflamm Bowel Dis. 2011;17:1751–8.
39. Karmiris K, Bielen D, Vanbeckevoort D, Vermeire S, Coremans G, Rutgeerts P, et al. Long-term monitoring of infliximab therapy for perianal fistulizing Crohn's disease by using magnetic resonance imaging. Clin Gastroenterol Hepatol. 2011;9:130–6.
40. Samaan MA, Puylaert CAJ, Levesque BG, Zou GY, Stitt L, Taylor SA, et al. The development of a magnetic resonance imaging index for fistulising Crohn's disease. Aliment Pharmacol Ther. 2017;46:516–28.
41. Pariente B, Mary J-Y, Danese S, Chowers Y, De Cruz P, D'Haens G, et al. Development of the Lémann index to assess digestive tract damage in patients with Crohn's disease. Gastroenterology. 2015;148:52–63.
42. Gilletta C, Lewin M, Bourrier A, Nion-Larmurier I, Rajca S, Beaugerie L, et al. Changes in the Lémann index values during the first years of Crohn's disease. Clin Gastroenterol Hepatol. 2015;13:1633–40.
43. Fiorino G, Bonifacio C, Allocca M, Repici A, Balzarini L, Malesci A, et al. Bowel damage as assessed by the Lémann index is reversible on anti-TNF therapy for Crohn's disease. J Crohns Colitis. 2015;9:633–9.
44. Fiorino G, Morin M, Bonovas S, Bonifacio C, Spinelli A, Germain A, et al. Prevalence of bowel damage assessed by cross-sectional imaging in early Crohn's disease and its impact on disease outcome. J Crohns Colitis. 2017;11:274–80.

MIX
Papier aus verantwortungsvollen Quellen
Paper from responsible sources
FSC® C105338

If you have any concerns about our products,
you can contact us on
ProductSafety@springernature.com

In case Publisher is established outside the EU,
the EU authorized representative is:
Springer Nature Customer Service Center GmbH
Europaplatz 3, 69115 Heidelberg, Germany

Printed by Libri Plureos GmbH
in Hamburg, Germany